Infectious Diseases
A Case Study Approach

Infectious Diseases
A Case Study Approach

Editor

Jonathan C. Cho, PharmD, MBA, BCIDP, BCPS

Clinical Associate Professor
Clinical Pharmacist, Infectious Diseases
Ben and Maytee Fisch College of Pharmacy
The University of Texas at Tyler
Tyler, Texas

New York   Chicago   San Francisco   Athens   London   Madrid   Mexico City
Milan   New Delhi   Singapore   Sydney   Toronto

Infectious Diseases: A Case Study Approach

1 2 3 4 5 6 7 8 9 LOV 25 24 23 22 21 20

ISBN 978-1-260-45510-6
MHID 1-260-45510-6

This book was set in Minion Pro by MPS Limited.
The editors were Michael Weitz and Peter J. Boyle.
The production supervisor was Catherine H. Saggese.
The text was designed by Alan Barnett.
Project management was provided by Touseen Qadri, MPS Limited.

This book is printed on acid-free paper.

Library of Congress Cataloging-in-Publication Data
Names: Cho, Jonathan C., editor.
Title: Infectious diseases : a case study approach / [edited by] Jonathan C. Cho.
Other titles: Infectious diseases (Cho)
Description: New York : McGraw Hill, [2020] | Includes bibliographical references and index.
Identifiers: LCCN 2019059148 (print) | LCCN 2019059149 (ebook) | ISBN 9781260455106
    (paperback) | ISBN 9781260455113 (ebook)
Subjects: MESH: Communicable Diseases—drug therapy | Communicable Diseases—diagnosis |
    Diagnosis, Differential | Case Reports | Problems and Exercises
Classification: LCC RC111 (print) | LCC RC111 (ebook) | NLM WC 18.2 | DDC 616.9—dc23
LC record available at https://lccn.loc.gov/2019059148
LC ebook record available at https://lccn.loc.gov/2019059149

CONTENTS

CONTRIBUTORS

Sean N. Avedissian, PharmD, MSc
Midwestern University Chicago College of Pharmacy, Downers Grove, Illinois
Northwestern Memorial Hospital, Department of Pharmacy, Chicago, Illinois
Chapter 5

Lisa Avery, PharmD, BCPS, BCIDP
Wegmans School of Pharmacy/St. John Fisher College, Rochester, New York
Chapter 32

P. Brandon Bookstaver, PharmD, BCPS
University of South Carolina College of Pharmacy, Columbia, South Carolina
Chapter 11

Elias B. Chahine, PharmD, BCPS, BCIDP
Palm Beach Atlantic University Lloyd L. Gregory School of Pharmacy, West Palm Beach, Florida
Chapter 26

Lindsey Childs-Kean, PharmD, MPH, BCPS
University of Florida College of Pharmacy, Gainesville, Florida
Chapter 24

Jonathan C. Cho, PharmD, MBA, BCIDP, BCPS
Department of Clinical Sciences
Ben and Maytee Fisch College of Pharmacy, University of Texas, Tyler, Texas
Chapters 4, 9, 17, 22, 27, 28, & 29

David Cluck, PharmD, BCPS, BCIDP, AAHIVP
East Tennessee State University–Gatton College of Pharmacy, Department of Pharmacy Practice, Johnson City, Tennessee
Chapter 34

Elizabeth A. Cook, PharmD, AE-C, BCACP, CDE
Ben and Maytee Fisch College of Pharmacy, University of Texas, Tyler, Texas
Chapter 28

Aimee Dassner, PharmD, BCIDP
Children's Health, Dallas, Texas
Chapter 2

Rebecca L. Dunn, PharmD, BCPS
Ben and Maytee Fisch College of Pharmacy, University of Texas, Tyler, Texas
Chapter 22

Rachel A. Foster, PharmD, MBA, BCIDP
Intermountain Healthcare, Murray, Utah
Chapter 11

Jason Gallagher, PharmD, BCPS
Temple University School of Pharmacy, Philadelphia, Pennsylvania
Chapter 1

Stephanie E. Giancola, PharmD, BCIDP, BCPS
Brooke Army Medical Center, Fort Sam Houston, Texas
Chapter 6

Amber B. Giles, PharmD, MPH, BCPS, AAHIVP
Presbyterian College School of Pharmacy, Clinton, South Carolina
Chapter 23

Jennifer E. Girotto, PharmD, BCPPS, BCIDP
University of Connecticut School of Pharmacy, Connecticut Children's Medical Center, Hartford, Connecticut
Chapter 2

Paul O. Gubbins, PharmD
University of Missouri – Kansas City, School of Pharmacy at Missouri State University, Springfield, Missouri
Chapter 30

Maria Heaney, PharmD
Temple University School of Pharmacy, Philadelphia, Pennsylvania
Chapter 1

Emily L. Heil, PharmD, BCIDP
University of Maryland School of Pharmacy, Baltimore, Maryland
Chapter 12

Elizabeth B. Hirsch, PharmD, BCPS
University of Minnesota College of Pharmacy, Minneapolis, Minneapolis
Chapter 6

Meghan N. Jeffres, PharmD, BCIDP
University of Colorado Skaggs School of Pharmacy and Pharmaceutical Sciences, Aurora, Colorado
Chapter 19

Michael Kelsch, PharmD, BCPS
North Dakota State University School of Pharmacy, Sanford Medical Center Fargo, Fargo, North Dakota
Chapter 15

Madeline King, PharmD, BCIDP
Philadelphia College of Pharmacy – University of the
Sciences, Philadelphia, Pennsylvania
Chapter 16

Wesley D. Kufel, PharmD, BCIDP, BCPS, AAHIVP
Binghamton University School of Pharmacy and
Pharmaceutical Sciences, State University of New York;
Upstate Medical University, State University of New York;
Upstate Medical University Hospital, Binghamton, New
York
Chapter 14

Ann Lloyd, PharmD, BCPS-AQ ID, BCIDP
The University of Oklahoma College of Pharmacy, Tulsa,
Oklahoma
Chapter 10

Jenana Maker, PharmD, BCPS
University of the Pacific Thomas J Long School of Pharmacy
and Health Sciences, Stockton, California
Chapter 3

Ashley H. Marx, PharmD, BCPS, BCIDP
University of North Carolina Eshelman School of Pharmacy,
Chapel Hill, North Carolina
Chapter 31

Jessica Robinson, PharmD, BCPS, BCIDP
University of Charleston School of Pharmacy, Charleston,
West Virginia
Chapter 33

Marc H. Scheetz, PharmD, MSc
Midwestern University Chicago College of Pharmacy,
Downers Grove, Illinois Northwestern Memorial Hospital,
Department of Pharmacy, Chicago, Illinois
Chapter 5

Kristy M. Shaeer, PharmD, MPH, BCIDP, AAHIVP
University of South Florida College of Pharmacy, Tampa,
Florida
Chapter 7

Elizabeth Sherman, PharmD, AAHIVP
Nova Southeastern University College of Pharmacy,
Memorial Healthcare System, Division of Infectious
Diseases, Southeast AIDS Education and Training Center,
Fort Lauderdale, Florida
Chapter 13

Winter J. Smith, PharmD, BCPS
Ben and Maytee Fisch College of Pharmacy, University
of Texas, Tyler, Texas
Chapter 29

Amelia K. Sofjan, PharmD, BCPS
University of Houston College of Pharmacy, Houston, Texas
Chapter 20

Kayla R. Stover, PharmD, BCIDP, BCPS
University of Mississippi School of Pharmacy, Jackson,
Mississippi
Chapter 18

Trent G. Towne, PharmD, BCPS
Manchester University College of Pharmacy, Natural
& Health Sciences, Fort Wayne, Indiana
Chapter 25

Jamie L. Wagner, PharmD, BCPS
University of Mississippi School of Pharmacy, Jackson,
Mississippi
Chapter 21

Takova D. Wallace-Gay, PharmD, BCACP
Ben and Maytee Fisch College of Pharmacy, University
of Texas, Tyler, Texas
Chapter 27

Jessica Wooster, PharmD, BCACP
Ben and Maytee Fisch College of Pharmacy, University
of Texas, Tyler, Texas
Chapter 28

Marylee V. Worley, PharmD, BCPS
Nova Southeastern University College of Pharmacy, Fort
Lauderdale, Florida
Chapter 8

Tianrui Yang, PharmD, BCPS
Ben and Maytee Fisch College of Pharmacy, University
of Texas, Tyler, Texas
Chapter 17

Frank S. Yu, PharmD
Ben and Maytee Fisch College of Pharmacy, University
of Texas, Tyler, Texas
Chapter 4

PREFACE

The goal of *Infectious Diseases: A Case Study Approach* is to provide healthcare students with a valuable infectious diseases pharmacotherapy resource. With the growing need of antimicrobial stewardship programs, healthcare professionals competent in infectious diseases pharmacotherapy are necessary.

This casebook is designed to teach infectious diseases through patient cases that closely resemble situations healthcare professionals will likely face during their clinical practice. Infectious diseases–related topics covered in this book range from bacterial infections, to sexually transmitted diseases, to antimicrobial dosing recommendations. Topics were selected based on the Accreditation Council for Pharmacy Education's Coding Systems for Colleges of Pharmacy and the 2016 American College of Clinical Pharmacy's Pharmacotherapy Didactic Curriculum Toolkit. Authors of this casebook chapters are comprised of infectious diseases pharmacist faculty from Colleges of pharmacy across the United States. All these individuals have vast experiences and training in infectious diseases and are widely recognized as experts in their field.

I hope that you will find this casebook useful during your studies!

Jonathan C. Cho, PharmD, MBA, BCIDP, BCPS
The University of Texas at Tyler
Tyler, Texas

1 Influenza

Maria Heaney   Jason Gallagher

PATIENT PRESENTATION

Chief Complaint

"I feel like I got hit by a truck. My body aches intensely, I'm weak, I have a fever, I'm lying under 3 blankets and can't get warm, and I can't stop shivering."

History of Present Illness

AW is a 34-year-old female presenting to the emergency department with a 2-day history of myalgia, chills, and fever to 102°F for which she has been using over-the-counter acetaminophen. She reports a rapid onset of symptoms, including nasal congestion and cough associated with chest pain. She denies a sore throat, but complains of nausea and vomiting that began a few weeks ago and has worsened acutely. She reports 3 episodes of emesis this morning prior to coming to the emergency department. She states she has never received the influenza vaccine, but all of her family members are vaccinated annually.

Past Medical History

Asthma, HTN, HLD, hypothyroidism

Surgical History

Appendectomy 6 years ago

Family History

Father has a history of MI; mother has HTN; sister has a history of breast cancer.

Social History

Married with 3 young, healthy children (ages 1, 3, and 6 years). Works as a 7th grade teacher. Denies illicit drug or tobacco use. Drinks alcohol socially.

Allergies

Penicillin (rash), egg (anaphylaxis)

Vaccines

UTD, refuses influenza vaccine due to egg allergy

Home Medications

Albuterol metered-dose inhaler 2 puffs q4h PRN shortness of breath

Amlodipine 10 mg PO daily

Atorvastatin 20 mg PO daily

Fluticasone-salmeterol 100 mcg/50 mcg 1 puff BID

Levothyroxine 112 mcg PO daily

Montelukast 10 mg PO QHS

Physical Examination

▶ Vital Signs

Temp 101.7°F, P 84, RR 18, BP 136/84 mm Hg, SaO$_2$ 97%, Ht 5′5″, Wt 64.5 kg

▶ General

Lethargic female with headache

▶ HEENT

Normocephalic, atraumatic, PERRLA, EOMI, pale/dry mucous membranes and conjunctiva

▶ Pulmonary

Stridorous breath sounds, equal lung expansion, cough present

▶ Cardiovascular

RRR, no murmurs, rubs, or gallops

▶ Abdomen

Soft, non-tender, non-distended, normoactive bowel sounds

▶ Genitourinary

Deferred

▶ Neurology

Lethargic, AAO ×3

▶ Extremities

Warm and well perfused, no edema

▶ Skin

No rashes, or lesions

Laboratory Findings

Na = 142 mEq/mL   Ca = 8.6 mg/dL   AST = 27 IU/L

K = 3.8 mEq/mL   Mg = 1.9 mg/dL   ALT = 19 IU/L

Cl = 98 mEq/mL   Phos = 3.6 mg/dL   T Bili = 0.5 mg/dL

CO_2 = 24 mEq/mL   Hgb = 15.1 mg/dL   Alk Phos = 36 IU/L

BUN = 17 mg/dL   Hct = 15.1 g/dL   Lactate = 0.7 mmol/L

SCr = 0.8 mg/dL   Plt = 184 × 10³/ mm³   hCG = 84,000 mIU/mL

Glu = 142 mg/dL   WBC = 8.2 × 10³/ mm³

QUESTIONS

1. Which of the following laboratory tests is the best option to assist in diagnosing AW in the emergency department?
   A. An influenza viral culture
   B. A rapid influenza cell culture
   C. A rapid influenza molecular assay
   D. A rapid influenza antigen detection test

2. Which of AW's symptoms and/or physical exam findings support a diagnosis of influenza?
   A. Rapid onset of fever and respiratory symptoms
   B. History of nausea and vomiting
   C. Body aches
   D. Both A and C

3. The influenza test performed for AW is positive for influenza A. Which of the following antiviral regimens is most appropriate to start?
   A. Baloxavir 20 mg PO once daily
   B. Amantadine 200 mg PO once daily
   C. Oseltamivir 75 mg PO BID
   D. Zanamivir 10 mg inhaled daily

4. What is the most appropriate duration of therapy for uncomplicated influenza treated with oseltamivir?
   A. 3 days
   B. 5 days
   C. 7 days
   D. 10 days

5. Which of the following adjunctive therapies should be added to AW's antiviral regimen?
   A. Methylprednisolone 60 mg IV daily
   B. IVIG 1 mg/kg IV once
   C. Piperacillin-tazobactam 3.375 g IV every 6 hours + vancomycin 1 g IV every 12 hours
   D. None of the above

6. Which of AW's family members should receive post-exposure chemoprophylaxis?
   A. Her 1-year-old child
   B. Her 3-year-old child

C. Both A and B
D. None of her family members should be offered chemoprophylaxis

7. Which of the following would be an appropriate chemoprophylaxis regimen for a patient with a CrCl of 80 to 85 mL/min?
   A. Oseltamivir 30 mg PO twice daily
   B. Peramivir 600 mg IV once
   C. Zanamivir 10 mg inhaled once daily
   D. Oseltamivir 30 mg PO once daily

8. Which of the following influenza vaccines is indicated for AW?
   A. Fluzone Quadrivalent
   B. Fluzone High-Dose
   C. FluMist Quadrivalent
   D. AW should not receive the influenza vaccine

9. Which of the following statements is true?
   A. Zanamivir is an acceptable alternative antiviral for treatment of influenza in AW
   B. AW should receive the influenza vaccine once treatment with an antiviral is initiated
   C. AW is at a relatively low risk for complications secondary to influenza infection
   D. Both A and B

ANSWERS

1. **Explanation:** The correct answer is C. Based on AW's presentation, it is likely that she has influenza. Influenza testing can have antimicrobial stewardship implications and can influence infection prevention and control decisions. During influenza season, outpatients and patients presenting to the emergency department should be tested for influenza if they present with acute-onset respiratory symptoms and are at high risk for complications secondary to influenza infection if the result may influence clinical management. Testing may be considered for patients who are not at high risk for complications if results may influence clinical management with regard to antiviral therapy, avoidance of unnecessary antibiotics or other diagnostic tests, and shortened time in the emergency department. Testing is recommended for all hospitalized patients during influenza season who have acute respiratory illness, have exacerbation of a chronic pulmonary or cardiac comorbidity, or are immunosuppressed with respiratory or other nonspecific symptoms. All of the above methods are reliable for detecting influenza. A rapid influenza cell culture has a high sensitivity and specificity; however, it takes 1 to 3 days to produce results which would not be ideal for rapid testing in the emergency department. While a viral culture has a high sensitivity and specificity, it takes 3 to 10 days for results. Since there are other testing methods available with a more rapid time to results, a viral culture is not the most efficient method for emergency department diagnostics.

The rapid molecular assay produces results in 15 to 20 minutes, and the rapid antigen detection test in 10 to 15 minutes. These methods are the most efficient for diagnosing influenza in the emergency department. Both methods have a high specificity, or the ability to detect a true negative result. The difference between the two is the sensitivity, or the ability to detect a true positive result. The rapid molecular assay detects influenza A or B viral RNA and has a high sensitivity, while the rapid antigen detection test has a low to moderate sensitivity and is not ideal for use in hospitalized patients. It is guideline recommended to use a rapid molecular assay over a rapid antigen detection test, when possible, to improve the detection of influenza infection.[1]

2. **Explanation:** The correct answer is D. Influenza is characterized by a rapid onset of respiratory symptoms, body aches, and exhaustion.[1] Though nausea and vomiting can be associated with influenza infection, this is not a typical presentation for adults. Additionally, AW has a several-week history of nausea, which is not a characteristic of influenza infection.

3. **Explanation:** The correct answer is C. Influenza treatment should be initiated promptly in patients with suspected or confirmed infection regardless of vaccination history if they are hospitalized, if they are outpatients with severe illness or at high risk of complications, including immuno-suppressed patients or those with chronic comorbidities, children <2 years old, adults 65 years or older, or women who are pregnant or within 2 weeks postpartum. Oseltamivir, peramivir, and zanamivir are all guideline-recommended agents for the treatment of influenza. Baloxavir is the most recently approved antiviral agent indicated for the treatment of uncomplicated influenza. This is not the correct answer choice because it is given as a single dose based on weight. For patients 40 to 80 kg, the dose is 40 mg once, and for patients ≥80 kg, the dose is 80 mg once. An important counseling point for baloxavir is that administration must be separated from polyvalent cations such as calcium, iron, and magnesium. Baloxavir is also not recommended for hospitalized patients with severe cases of influenza due to a lack of data in this population.[2] Zanamivir 10 mg inhaled daily is a chemoprophylaxis dose. The treatment dose of zanamivir is 10 mg inhaled twice daily. Additionally, there is limited data for the use of inhaled zanamivir in hospitalized patients with severe cases of influenza, and this is not a preferred agent in pregnancy due to concern for lower lung volumes which may result in reduced drug exposure and bronchospasm. Adamantane antivirals such as amantadine are no longer recommended due to viral resistance. Oseltamivir is the preferred antiviral in hospitalized patients, as well as in pregnancy.[1]

4. **Explanation:** The correct answer is B. According to the guideline recommendations and FDA approval, immunocompetent adults with influenza should receive a 5-day course when being treated with oseltamivir. In certain situations, such as in immunocompromised patients with severe influenza infection, a 10-day course may be considered. Critical illness is another scenario in which a longer duration of treatment may be considered, though there is no well-defined duration in this population.[1] AW is not immunocompromised, nor is she critically ill, thus a 5-day course of therapy is adequate to treat her influenza.

5. **Explanation:** The correct answer is D. Corticosteroid administration in patients with influenza has been associated with increased mortality in hospitalized patients in observational studies and is not recommended for adjunctive therapy. Immunotherapy, such as with IVIG, can have immune modulating effects and neutralize viral activity; however, significant clinical benefit over antiviral agents has not yet been determined in clinical study. IVIG should not routinely be used as adjunctive therapy. Lastly, piperacillin-tazobactam is an antibacterial agent. Bacterial coinfection is possible in patients with influenza, and may be present upon initial influenza diagnosis or may manifest later and result in clinical deterioration. Bacterial coinfection should be investigated and empirically treated in patients presenting with severe disease consisting of extensive pneumonia on imaging, respiratory failure, hypotension, and fever. Bacterial coinfection may also be considered in patients who deteriorate after initial improvement on an antiviral agent or in those who fail to improve within 3 to 5 days of antiviral therapy. In patients with severe bacterial pneumonia complicating influenza, *Staphylococcus aureus*, including MRSA, accounts for many cases, thus an anti-MRSA antibiotic should be included in empiric bacterial coverage in such cases.[1] For AW, antibiotics are not required for adjunctive therapy because her presenting symptoms did not include evidence of severe pneumonia, respiratory failure, or hypotension.

6. **Explanation:** The correct answer is D. Post-exposure chemoprophylaxis with antivirals is not recommended routinely, but may be considered in certain patient populations. Chemoprophylaxis may be administered to adults and children ≥3 months old at high risk of complications from influenza, such as patients who are severely immunocompromised and for whom vaccination is contraindicated. If adults and children ≥3 months old are exposed to influenza and are household contacts of an immunocompromised patient, it is recommended that chemoprophylaxis is administered for 7 days after exposure along with the inactivated influenza vaccine. Patients exposed to influenza who do not receive chemoprophylaxis should be monitored closely and treated promptly if symptoms develop, especially those at high risk for complications from infection, including children <5 years old (and especially <2 years old), elderly patients ≥65 years old, women who are pregnant or postpartum, morbidly obese patients, nursing home residents, and patients with chronic pulmonary, cardiac, or metabolic diseases.[1] Pre-exposure

chemoprophylaxis with oseltamivir or zanamivir may also be considered in patients ≥3 months old at high risk for complications, including aforementioned populations as well as hematopoietic stem cell transplants recipients within 6 to 12 months posttransplant and lung transplant recipients. Pre-exposure chemoprophylaxis is given for the duration of influenza season in most cases.[1] AW reported that all members of her family are healthy and have received the influenza vaccine, thus post-exposure chemoprophylaxis is not indicated in this situation. Her 1-year-old and 3-year-old children, however, should be very closely monitored for symptoms as they are at high risk for complications from influenza.

7. **Explanation:** The correct answer is C. The chemoprophylaxis dose of oseltamivir is 75 mg PO once daily for patients with normal renal function. Oseltamivir 30 mg PO twice daily is a renally adjusted treatment dose, and 30 mg PO once daily is a renally adjusted dose that can be used for treatment or prophylaxis. Peramivir is not indicated for chemoprophylaxis. Pre-exposure prophylaxis is given for the duration of influenza activity in the community in most cases, whereas post-exposure chemoprophylaxis is given for 7 days after the initial influenza exposure.[1]

8. **Explanation:** The correct answer is A. Fluzone High-Dose is an inactivated influenza vaccine indicated for patients ≥65 years. FluMist Quadrivalent is a live attenuated influenza vaccine (LAIV).[3] An egg allergy of any severity is no longer a contraindication to LAIV administration and is listed as safe for administration by the Advisory Committee on Immunization Practices (ACIP). For AW, however, we would avoid the use of the LAIV because it is not recommended for administration to pregnant women according to ACIP.[4]

9. **Explanation:** The correct answer is B. Since AW is pregnant as evidenced by her elevated hCG, she is at high risk for complications secondary to influenza, including cardiopulmonary disease, premature labor, and fetal loss. Chronic pulmonary disease, including asthma, also puts patients at a higher risk for complications.[1] Patients, especially pregnant women and others at higher risk for complications, should receive the influenza vaccine even if they are infected with influenza in order to protect against other influenza strains and future infection. According to the CDC, it is acceptable to administer an inactivated influenza vaccine during treatment with an antiviral. Live attenuated influenza vaccines should be avoided until 48 hours after completing therapy with an antiviral.[5] In pregnancy, inhaled zanamivir is not preferred for treatment due to concern for reduced drug distribution and bronchospasm resulting from lower lug volumes. Zanamivir is also not recommended for use in patients with respiratory disease, including asthma. Oseltamivir is the preferred agent for treatment in pregnancy.[1]

REFERENCES

1. Uyeki TM, Bernstein HH, Bradley JS, et al. Clinical practice guidelines by the Infectious Diseases Society of America: 2018 update on diagnosis, treatment, chemoprophylaxis, and institutional outbreak management of seasonal influenza. *Clin Infect Dis.* 2018;68(6):e1–e47.

2. Baloxavir marboxil [package insert]. San Francisco, CA: Genentech USA, Inc.; 2018. Available at https://www.gene.com/download/pdf/xofluza_prescribing.pdf. Accessed April 18, 2019.

3. Centers for Disease Control and Prevention. Recommended immunization schedule for adults aged 19 years or older, United States, 2018. Available at https://www.cdc.gov/vaccines/schedules/hcp/imz/adult.html. Accessed February 7, 2019.

4. Grohskopf LA, Sokolow LZ, Broder KR, Walter EB, Fry AM, Jernigan DB. Prevention and control of seasonal influenza with vaccines: Recommendations of the Advisory Committee on Immunization Practices-United States, 2018–19 influenza season. *MMWR Recomm Rep.* 2018;67(3):1-20.

5. Centers for Disease Control and Prevention. Influenza vaccination: A summary for clinicians. CDC Web site. Available at https://www.cdc.gov/flu/professionals/vaccination/vax-summary.htm. Accessed April 18, 2019.

2 Acute Otitis Media

Aimee Dassner   Jennifer E. Girotto

PATIENT PRESENTATION

Chief Complaint

"Increased irritability and right ear pain."

History of Present Illness

JL is a 22-month-old female who presents to her primary care provider (PCP) with a 2-day history of rhinorrhea and a 1-day history of increased irritability, fever (to 101.5°F per Mom), and right-ear tugging. Mom denies that JL has had any nausea, vomiting, or diarrhea.

Past Medical History

Full-term birth via spontaneous vaginal delivery. Hospitalized at 9 months of age for respiratory syncytial virus–associated bronchiolitis. Two episodes of acute otitis media (AOM), with last episode about 6 months earlier.

Surgical History

None

Social History

Lives with mother, father, and her 5-year-old brother who attends kindergarten. JL attends daycare 2 d/wk, and stays at home with maternal grandmother 3 d/wk.

Allergies

No known drug allergies

Immunizations

Immunization	Age Administered
Hepatitis B	Birth
DTap/Hep B/IPV	2 mo, 4 mo, 6 mo
Hib	2 mo, 4 mo, 6 mo, 15 mo
PCV13	2 mo, 4 mo, 6 mo, 12 mo
Influenza	6 mo, 8 mo, 18 mo
MMR	12 mo
Varicella	12 mo

Home Medications

Vitamin D drops 600 IU/d

Physical Examination

▶ **Vital Signs (while crying)**

Temp 100.7°F, P 140 bpm, RR 35, BP 100/57 mm Hg, Ht 81 cm, Wt 23.7 kg

▶ **General**

Fussy, but consolable by Mom; well-appearing

▶ **HEENT**

Normocephalic, atraumatic, moist mucous membranes, normal conjunctiva, clear rhinorrhea, moderate bulging and erythema of right tympanic membrane with middle-ear effusion

▶ **Pulmonary**

Good air movement throughout, clear breath sounds bilaterally

▶ **Cardiovascular**

Normal rate and rhythm, no murmur, rub or gallop

▶ **Abdomen**

Soft, non-distended, non-tender, active bowel sounds

▶ **Genitourinary**

Normal female genitalia, no dysuria or hematuria

▶ **Neurology**

Alert and appropriate for age

▶ **Extremities**

Normal

QUESTIONS

1. Which of the following clinical criteria is *not* part of the diagnostic evaluation or staging of acute otitis media (AOM) for this patient?
   A. Rhinorrhea
   B. Fever
   C. Otalgia
   D. Contour of the tympanic membrane

2. Which of the following is a risk factor for AOM?
   A. Vaginal delivery
   B. History of RSV at 9 months

C. Day care attendance

D. Immunizations up to date

3. Which of the following best describes the clinical presentation of AOM for this patient?

A. Non-severe, bilateral

B. Non-severe, unilateral

C. Severe, bilateral

D. Severe, unilateral

4. What is the recommended management for AOM in this patient?

A. Culture the middle ear fluid, then treat with culture-directed antibiotics

B. Acetaminophen 15 mg/kg PO q6h, with patient follow-up in 2 to 3 days

C. Acetaminophen 15 mg/kg PO q6h PRN and amoxicillin 45 mg/kg PO q12h

D. Acetaminophen 15 mg/kg PO q6h PRN and cefdinir 14 mg/kg PO q24h

E. Acetaminophen 15 mg/kg PO q6h PRN and amoxicillin/clavulanate 30 mg/kg q8h

5. Forty-eight hours after initial presentation, the patient's mother calls the PCP to report persistent otalgia and fevers (T_{max} 102°F), with complaints of new-onset left ear pain. Which of the following would be the most appropriate antimicrobial therapy to start for this patient?

A. Amoxicillin

B. Amoxicillin/clavulanate

C. Cefdinir

D. Azithromycin

6. You have recommended that JL be prescribed amoxicillin at a dose of 30 mg/kg/dose q8h. The community pharmacist calls and asks to verify if this dose is correct or if 45 mg/kg/dose q12h would be better. Which of the following would be a reason that you would prefer the 30 mg/kg/dose q8h over a dose of 45 mg/kg/dose q12h?

A. Increased rates of *H. influenzae* resistance in your community

B. Increased rates of oral penicillin non-susceptible pneumococci in your community

C. Increased rates of *M. catarrhalis* in your community

D. There is no reason that 30 mg/kg/dose q8h would be preferred

7. What is the appropriate duration of antibiotic therapy for treatment of AOM for JL?

A. 5 days

B. 7 days

C. 10 days

D. 14 days

8. Per the current AAP guidelines for the diagnosis and management of acute otitis media, which of the following routinely administered pediatric vaccine(s) is/are recommended by the AAP to help prevent AOM in infants and children?

A. Pneumococcal conjugate vaccine (PCV13)

B. *H. influenzae* type b (Hib)

C. Influenza (Flu)

D. Both A and C

E. All of the above

9. If JL continued to have multiple episodes of AOM, prophylactic antibiotics should be considered to reduce the frequency of AOM episodes in which of the following situations:

A. 3 episodes of AOM in 6 months

B. 4 episodes of AOM in 1 year

C. 6 episodes of AOM in 2 years

D. Never

ANSWERS

1. **Explanation:** The correct answer is A. Per the 2013 American Academy of Pediatrics (AAP) guidelines for "The Diagnosis and Management of Acute Otitis Media,"[1] clinical criteria for the diagnosis and severity staging (non-severe versus severe) of AOM include otorrhea, otalgia, fever, visualization of tympanic membrane (TM) contour (normal, mild bulging, moderate bulging or severe bulging) and color, and presence of middle ear effusion (MEE). AOM should not be diagnosed in patients without MEE. Additionally, a moderate to severe bulging TM is the most important clinical sign in the diagnosis of AOM, and has been highly associated with bacterial etiology of infection.

2. **Explanation:** The correct answer is C. Day care attendance is a well-known risk factor for AOM. Other risk factors for AOM is a family member with AOM, parental smoking, and pacifier usage.[2]

3. **Explanation:** The correct answer is B. This patient only has complaints and signs of otalgia in the right ear, which would make this a unilateral presentation of AOM. Severe AOM is defined as a toxic-appearing child, or persistent otalgia >48 hours, or a temperature ≥39°C (102.2°F) in the past 48 hours. This patient does not meet any of these criteria.[1]

4. **Explanation:** The correct answer is B. All children with AOM and otalgia should be offered pain management, so acetaminophen (an analgesic and antipyretic) is appropriate to prescribe for this patient. Both viral and bacterial pathogens can cause AOM, but identification of causative pathogens is not routinely performed for non-refractory AOM in clinical practice.[1,3] The majority of AOM episodes are viral in origin and are self-limiting, as are many types of bacterial AOM. Pneumococcal AOM is the least likely bacterial AOM to resolve on its own. Severe AOM, AOM in patients <6 months and non-severe bilateral AOM in young patients (6 to 24 months) have been most often associated with increased rates of clinical failure. Patients without these criteria are generally recommended to have an initial period of observation prior to antibiotic prescribing. If AOM worsens or does not improve after 48 to 72 hours of observation, a bacterial

etiology that is unlikely to self-resolve can be presumed and antibiotics should be prescribed. AAP guideline recommendations for approach to initial management of AOM in children are summarized in Table 2.1, adapted from AAP guidelines.[1]

5. **Explanation:** The correct answer is A. The most common bacterial pathogens in AOM are *Streptococcus pneumoniae*, non-typeable *Haemophilus influenzae,* and *Moraxella catarrhalis*. The causative etiology of bacterial AOM has shifted since the onset of routine pneumococcal vaccination with PCV7 in 2000, and its subsequent replacement with PCV13 in 2010. Specifically, the prevalence of circulating penicillin-resistant *S. pneumoniae* strains has decreased.

   When properly dosed, amoxicillin (90 mg/kg/d as q8h dosing) can provide adequate time above the minimum inhibitory concentration (MIC) for *S. pneumoniae* isolates with a penicillin MIC ≤2 µg/mL (current susceptibility breakpoint). The addition of clavulanate to amoxicillin (amoxicillin/clavulanate) provides additional coverage against beta-lactamase-producing organisms, but does *not* provide any additional coverage against resistant *S. pneumoniae* over amoxicillin. Although 18% to 42% of *H. influenzae* and 100% of *M. catarrhalis* isolates produce beta-lactamase, 48% to 75% of AOM infections with these organisms, respectively, are self-limiting. Therefore, high-dose amoxicillin (90 mg/kg/d) is recommended as first-line treatment for antibiotic-naive (no antibiotics within 30 days) patients as a narrow-spectrum, affordable antibiotic with minimal adverse effects.[1] Amoxicillin/clavulanate is recommended for AOM treatment only in the following situations: if a patient presents with concurrent bilateral conjunctivitis (suggestive of *H. influenzae*

infection), if they have received antibiotics in the past 30 days, or if they fail initial therapy with amoxicillin.[1]

Cefdinir is listed in the AAP guidelines as an alternative first-line treatment for penicillin-allergic patients.[1] However, it is important to note that cefdinir has decreased empiric in vitro *S. pneumoniae* susceptibilities compared to amoxicillin (70% to 80% versus 84% to 92% susceptible). Lastly, azithromycin is not recommended for AOM, due to poor activity against both *S. pneumoniae* and *H. influenzae*.[1]

6. **Explanation:** The correct answer is B. Change of the dose of amoxicillin from q12h to q8h improves the time above the MIC up until an MIC of approximately 2 µg/mL.[3] Since both *H. influenzae* and *M. catarrhalis* produce beta-lactamase, a switch to amoxicillin/clavulanate would be most appropriate instead of a change in dose.

7. **Explanation:** The correct answer is C. While the optimal duration of therapy for AOM is unknown, 10 days of antibiotics is the current standard duration of therapy. Several studies have evaluated shorter courses of antibiotics for treatment of AOM, with results suggesting that 7 and 5 days of antibiotic therapy may be equally as effective as 10 days in children aged 2 to 5 years and ≥6 years with mild to moderate AOM, respectively.[1] However, JL is not yet 2 years old, so these shorter treatment courses would not be appropriate. Notably, a 2016 *New England Journal of Medicine* article evaluating a 5-day versus 10-day course of amoxicillin/clavulanate for the treatment of AOM in children 6 to 23 months of age found that children treated with 5 days of antibiotics were more likely to experience clinical failure.[4]

8. **Explanation:** The correct answer is D. AAP guidelines recommend vaccination with the pneumococcal conjugate and influenza vaccines according to the schedule set forth by the Advisory Committee on Immunization Practices for the prevention of AOM in all children.[1] Note that although the bacteria *H. influenzae* is associated with AOM, type b *H. influenzae* was associated more with systemic disease (eg, epiglottitis, pneumonia) as opposed to AOM.

9. **Explanation:** The correct answer is D. Current AAP guidelines recommend against the use of antimicrobial prophylaxis for the prevention of recurrent AOM in children.[1] The potential small benefit of antimicrobial prophylaxis for AOM does not outweigh the risks of adverse effects from antibiotics, effects of prolonged antibiotic use on increasing antimicrobial resistance, and additional cost to patient families. Patients who experience recurrent AOM (defined as 3 episodes in 6 months or 4 episodes in 1 year) are candidates for tympanostomy tube placement.

REFERENCES

1. Lieberthal AS, Carroll AE, Chonmaitree T, et al. The diagnosis and management of acute otitis media. *Pediatrics.* 2013;131:e964-e999.

TABLE 2.1. Recommendations for Initial Management of AOM

Presentation	Age	Antibiotics	Pain Management
Severe, Unilateral or Bilateral	Any	YES	YES
Non-severe, Unilateral	<6 months	YES	YES
	≥6 months	Additional Observation[a]	
Non-severe, Bilateral	<24 months	YES	YES
	≥24 months	Additional Observation[a]	

[a]The decision to manage with additional observation should be made in conjunction with the patient's family and follow-up should be ensured at 48 to 72 hours. Antibiotics should be initiated if the child worsens, or fails to improve within 48 to 72 hours.
Source: Adapted from reference 1.

2. Uhari M, Mantysaari K, Niemela M. A meta-analytic review of the risk factors for acute otitis media. *Clin Infect Dis*. 1996;22(6):1079-1083.

3. Fallon RM, Kuti JL, Doern GV, et al. Pharmacodynamic target attainment of oral β-lactams for the empiric treatment of acute otitis media in children. *Pediatr Drugs*. 2008;10(5):329-335.

4. Hoberman A, Paradise JL, Rockette HE, et al. Shortened antimicrobial treatment for acute otitis media in young children. *N Engl J Med*. 2016;375(25):2446-2456.

3 Acute Bronchitis

Jenana Maker

PATIENT PRESENTATION

Chief Complaint

"I can't stop coughing."

History of Present Illness

MT is a 35-year-old female who presents to her primary care physician with cough for the last 10 days. She explains that her 6-year-old son had fever, runny nose, and cough about 2 weeks ago but got better after a few days. She explains that she got sick shortly after him and developed nasal congestion, sore throat, and a productive cough. While her congestion has improved, she continues to cough and is concerned that her symptoms still persist. She denies any fever, chills, dyspnea, or hemoptysis.

Past Medical History

Hypothyroidism, insomnia

Surgical History

None

Family History

Father has HTN and hyperlipidemia, mother has history of breast cancer and is in remission. One younger sister (age 30), who is alive and well.

Social History

Married with two children (ages 6 and 8), works as a dental hygienist, denies smoking and illicit drug use

Allergies

NKDA

Home Medications

Levothyroxine 50 mcg orally once daily
Alprazolam 0.25 mg orally nightly as needed for insomnia

Physical Examination

▶ Vital Signs

Temp 98.8°F, P 68, RR 16, BP 115/73 mm Hg, O_2 saturation 98%, Ht 5′9″, Wt 63 kg

▶ General

Well-developed female in NAD

▶ HEENT

PERRLA, EOMI, TMs intact, moist mucous membranes, mild pharyngeal erythema present

▶ Neck/Lymph Nodes

Supple, no lymphadenopathy

▶ Pulmonary

CTA, no crackles/wheezing, cough present

▶ Cardiovascular

NSR, no m/r/g

▶ Abdomen

Soft, non-tender, non-distended, bowel sounds present

▶ Genitourinary

Deferred

▶ Neurology

A&O ×3, CN intact

▶ MS/Extremities

Deferred

Laboratory Findings

Na = 136 mEq/L	Hgb = 14 g/dL
K = 3.9 mEq/L	Hct = 40%
Cl = 100 mEq/L	Plt = 201 × 10³/mm³
CO_2 = 22 mEq/L	WBC = 9 × 10³/mm³
BUN = 12 mg/dL	
Scr = 0.8 mg/dL	
Glu = 98 mg/dL	

▶ Rapid Influenza Test

Negative

QUESTIONS

1. Which of the following is a hallmark symptom of acute bronchitis?
   A. Cough
   B. Fever
   C. Sputum production
   D. Nasal congestion

2. Which of the following clinical or laboratory parameters is needed to establish the diagnosis of acute bronchitis in this patient?
   A. Sputum culture
   B. Chest X-ray
   C. Patient's clinical presentation and physical exam
   D. Spirometry testing

3. Which of the following microorganisms is the most likely pathogen responsible for MT's symptoms?
   A. *Streptococcus pneumoniae*
   B. *Mycoplasma pneumoniae*
   C. *Bordetella pertussis*
   D. Respiratory viruses

4. Which of the following antimicrobials would be most appropriate to recommend for MT?
   A. Amoxicillin/clavulanic acid 875/125 mg orally twice daily
   B. Azithromycin 500 mg orally once, then 250 mg orally once daily
   C. Oseltamivir 75 mg orally twice daily
   D. Antimicrobial therapy is not recommended for MT

5. Which of the following over-the-counter therapies may be most helpful in alleviating MT's symptoms?
   A. Albuterol
   B. Dextromethorphan
   C. Pseudoephedrine
   D. Diphenhydramine

6. What is the desired goal of MT's pharmacotherapeutic plan?
   A. Resolution of cough
   B. Eradication of infection
   C. Preventing hospitalization
   D. Preventing spread of infection into the bloodstream and/or other organs

7. Which of the following conditions is typically *present* in patients with chronic bronchitis but *absent* in patients with acute bronchitis?
   A. Presence of purulent sputum production
   B. Past medical history of smoking
   C. Past medical history of multiple respiratory infections
   D. Presence of reversible airflow limitation on spirometry testing

ANSWERS

1. **Explanation:** The correct answer is A. Cough is the hallmark feature of acute bronchitis and tends to persist for multiple days and up to 3 weeks. In addition to cough, patients may experience sputum production with or without purulence. Further, some patients may experience mild dyspnea, wheezing, and bronchial hyperresponsiveness. As cough persists, some patients may complain of substernal or chest wall pain when coughing. Fever is rarely present in patients with acute bronchitis and typically indicates influenza or pneumonia (rules out Answer B). Sputum production and nasal congestion may or may not be present (rules out Answers C and D).[1,2]

2. **Explanation:** The correct answer is C. The diagnosis of acute bronchitis is typically established with a physical exam and patient's clinical presentation. Specifically, her findings of a persistent cough and sputum production are indicative of acute bronchitis. A sputum culture is typically not indicated as bacteria are rarely implicated in acute bronchitis (rules out Answer A). Chest X-ray is typically reserved for patients with signs/symptoms suspicious of pneumonia (rules out Answer B). Spirometry testing is not indicated and is largely used in patients with chronic respiratory conditions such as asthma, COPD, or interstitial lung disease (rules out Answer D).[1,2]

3. **Explanation:** The correct answer is D. Respiratory viruses account for 85% to 95% of all acute bronchitis cases. The most commonly isolated viruses include rhinovirus, influenza A and B, parainfluenza, respiratory syncytial virus, and coronavirus. Of note, patients who test positive for influenza virus in the setting of fever and cough may need to be further evaluated for treatment with antiviral therapy. Fewer than 10% of cases are caused by atypical bacteria such as *Bordetella pertussis, Chlamydophila pneumoniae*, or *Mycoplasma pneumoniae* (rules out Answers A, B, C).[3]

4. **Explanation:** The correct answer is D. Antibiotics such as amoxicillin/clavulanic acid and azithromycin are not recommended since bacteria rarely cause acute bronchitis (rules out Answers A and B). Oseltamivir is an antiviral but, since it is only active against the influenza virus, it would not be recommended for this patient (Answer C is incorrect). There is limited evidence of clinical benefit to support the use of antibiotics in acute bronchitis. Studies indicate that antibiotics only modestly reduce severity and duration of symptoms (eg, duration or cough and impaired activity are reduced by only a fraction of a day). On the other hand, antibiotic use can increase risk of antimicrobial resistance, antibiotic-related adverse effects, and treatment cost. Still, it is estimated that 70% to 90% of patients with acute bronchitis receive a prescription for an antiviral or antibiotic agent. Antimicrobial therapy should be reserved for cases where a bacterial pathogen is isolated or in high-risk patients presenting with symptoms of influenza during influenza season. If treatment is needed, the duration of antimicrobial therapy depends somewhat on the antimicrobial agent but is typically between 5 and 10 days.[3,4]

5. **Explanation:** The correct answer is B. Dextromethorphan may help this patient by relieving her cough symptoms.

Another reasonable option would be an expectorant such as guaifenesin that has been shown to significantly reduce cough frequency and sputum thickness when compared to placebo. Short-acting β_2 agonists such as albuterol have been found to only be beneficial in patients with bronchial hyperresponsiveness or wheezing upon presentation as well as patients with evidence of airway obstruction. Since MT has no evidence of wheezing or airway obstruction, albuterol would not be indicated (rules out Answer A). Further, a nasal decongestant such as pseudoephedrine would also not be indicated since the patient's congestion has improved on its own (rules out Answer C). Lastly, there is no indication for an antihistamine such as diphenhydramine (rules out Answer D).[2-4]

6. **Explanation:** The correct answer is A. Persistent cough is the chief complaint for this patient and can be managed with supportive therapies such as over-the-counter medications. Since the infection is caused by respiratory viruses, no antimicrobial treatment for the infection is available to eradicate it (rules out Answer B). The patient's infection is mild and her age and lack of serious comorbidities put her at a very low risk for hospitalization (rules out Answer C). Acute bronchitis is typically limited to the respiratory tract with no risk for dissemination (rules out Answer D).

7. **Explanation:** The correct answer is B. Chronic bronchitis is broadly defined as presence of cough and sputum production lasting for 3 months or longer for two consecutive years or more. Chronic bronchitis is caused by chronic exposure to cigarette smoke or other noxious agents and is typically associated with chronic obstructive pulmonary disease (COPD). In contrast to acute bronchitis, it is typically not curable but patients can slow down disease progression with appropriate lifestyle modifications, particularly smoking cessation. Patients with COPD and chronic bronchitis are at an increased risk for COPD exacerbations which, in contrast to acute bronchitis, are usually precipitated by an infection. The most common organisms associated with COPD exacerbations are *Haemophilus influenzae, Moraxella catarrhalis, Streptococcus pneumoniae,* and *Haemophilus parainfluenzae.* Treatment with antibiotics is indicated if the patient has increased dyspnea, sputum volume, and sputum purulence, or requires mechanical ventilation. Antibiotics for COPD exacerbations have been shown to decrease length of hospitalization, recovery time, and treatment failure. Purulent sputum production may be present in both acute and chronic bronchitis (rules out Answer A). Past medical history of respiratory infections varies widely between patients and is not a recommended parameter to distinguish acute and chronic bronchitis (rules out Answer C). Presence of reversible airflow limitation on spirometry testing is typically associated with asthma (rules out Answer D).[5]

REFERENCES

1. Blackford MG, Glover ML, Reed MD. Lower respiratory tract infections. In: DiPiro JT, Talbert RL, Yee GC, Matzke GR, Wells BG, Posey L, eds. *Pharmacotherapy: A Pathophysiologic Approach.* 10ed. New York, NY: McGraw-Hill.

2. Kinkade S, Long NA. Acute bronchitis. *Am Fam Physician.* 2016;94(7):560-565.

3. Smith SM, Fahey T, Smucny J, Becker LA. Antibiotics for acute bronchitis. *Cochrane Database Syst Rev.* 2017;6:CD000245.

4. Tackett KL, Atkins A. Evidence-based acute bronchitis therapy. *J Pharm Prac.* 2012;25(6):586-590.

5. Global Initiative for Chronic Obstructive Lung Disease. Global strategy for the diagnosis, management, and prevention of chronic obstructive lung disease 2019 report. Available at https://goldcopd.org/wp-content/uploads/2018/11/GOLD-2019-v1.7-FINAL-14Nov2018-WMS.pdf. Accessed April 24, 2019.

4 Pharyngitis

Frank S. Yu   Jonathan C. Cho

PATIENT PRESENTATION

Chief Complaint

"Mommy, my throat is on fire!"

History of Present Illness

JT is a 7-year-old Chinese American female, accompanied by her mother, who presents to the community pharmacy with complaints of sore throat and fever, looking for medications to take to relieve her symptoms. She is fussy and describes the pain when she swallows as feeling if her throat is "on fire." Her symptoms began yesterday morning, and she has only tried drinking a pei pa koa syrup containing medicinal herbs (main active herb is elm bark) and honey to relieve the sore throat. This provided some relief but the pain has been getting worse. She did not have a temperature taken, but her forehead was hot to the touch. She was not given any medications to relieve the fever. She was dressed with additional clothing and blankets to "sweat the fever out," but the fever still persisted. She reports that there may have been other sick classmates. She denies a prior history of sore throat.

Past Medical History

Attention-deficit disorder, recurrent otitis media (resolved)

Surgical History

None

Family History

Non-contributory

Social History

Ear tubes at age 2

Allergies

Amoxicillin (throat swelling, difficulty breathing)

Home Medications

Methylphenidate ER 18 mg PO daily

Physical Examination

▸ Vital Signs

Temp 101.9°F (oral), Ht 4′4″, Wt 29.55 kg

▸ General

Appears uncomfortable, tired, grimacing when swallowing

▸ HEENT

Anterior cervical lymph nodes enlarged and tender; tonsils moist, red, with white exudates

▸ Point-of-Care GAS Rapid Antigen Detection Test

Positive

QUESTIONS

1. What is the most common pathogen responsible for acute bacterial pharyngitis in children?
   A. *Corynebacterium diphtheriae*
   B. *Neisseria gonorrhoeae*
   C. Group C streptococcus
   D. Group A streptococcus

2. What signs and symptoms in this patient definitely discriminate between GAS pharyngitis rather than viral pharyngitis?
   A. Tonsils with white exudates
   B. Temperature 101.9°F
   C. Pain on swallowing
   D. All of the above

3. If GAS is suspected, what age range is typically excluded for testing for GAS?
   A. Age <3 years
   B. Age 5–15 years
   C. Age 16–64 years
   D. Age >65 years

4. Which of the following antibiotic treatment regimens should be recommended for JT based on patient-specific factors and general resistance patterns?
   A. Cephalexin 500 mg orally twice daily × 10 days
   B. Clindamycin 207 mg orally three times daily × 10 days
   C. Azithromycin 354 mg orally once daily × 5 days
   D. Clarithromycin 222 mg orally twice daily × 10 days

5. Which of the following counseling points is not true for the medication selected above?
   A. Store the medication in the refrigerator
   B. Rash
   C. Diarrhea
   D. Badly tasting medication

6. JT's parent asks what else can be given to help with her child's discomfort. What do you recommend?
   A. Aspirin 81 mg orally every 4 to 6 hours as needed for fever or pain
   B. Prednisolone 15 mg orally twice daily
   C. Acetaminophen 400 mg orally every 4 to 6 hours as needed for fever or pain
   D. All of the above

7. JT presents back to your pharmacy two more times with complaints of sore throat, cough, raspy voice, and positive GAS RADT over the next 12 months. What is the most likely cause of these recurrent cases of GAS pharyngitis?
   A. Recurrent viral infections, with falsely identified GAS presence
   B. Inadequate antimicrobial therapy due to medication noncompliance
   C. Recurrent viral infections, while carrying GAS
   D. New infections from different GAS strains

8. JT's parent asks if JT should get her tonsils taken out to prevent this from occurring again in the future. What do you recommend?
   A. Yes
   B. No

ANSWERS

1. **Explanation:** The correct answer is D. Group A streptococcus (GAS, most commonly *Streptococcus pyogenes*) is the most common pathogen responsible for acute bacterial pharyngitis in children. *C. diphtheriae* and *N. gonorrhoeae* can cause acute bacterial pharyngitis and can be treated by antimicrobial therapy, but are rare. Group C streptococcus is a common cause of acute bacterial pharyngitis in college students and adults, but not usually present in children. However, viruses such as adenovirus, influenza virus, parainfluenza virus, and rhinovirus are the most common causes of acute pharyngitis cases in general.[1] GAS is the only pathogen that generally warrants antibiotic therapy because pharyngitis due to other organisms has no proven benefit. Preventing the exposure of patients to unnecessary antimicrobial therapy due to non-GAS pharyngitis is good antimicrobial stewardship practice to reduce cost, adverse effects, and resistance. Appropriate treatment and eradication of GAS reduce the development of other conditions such as acute rheumatic fever with or without carditis, and post-streptococcal glomerulonephritis.[1]

2. **Explanation:** The correct answer is D. Patients with GAS typically present with sudden-onset sore throat, pain on swallowing, and fever. Children may also develop headache, nausea, vomiting, and abdominal pain. Tonsillopharyngeal erythema with or without exudates, and tender, enlarged anterior cervical lymph nodes are usually present on physical examination. Absence of fever, conjunctivitis, coryza/rhinorrhea, cough, oral ulcers, discrete ulcerative stomatitis, hoarseness, and viral exanthema are more suggestive of viral pharyngitis.[1] Clinical signs and symptoms of pharyngitis may overlap between GAS pharyngitis and viral pharyngitis, so diagnosis based on features alone is less accurate. Previous literature referred to scoring systems such as CENTOR to establish probability of GAS pharyngitis, but that is no longer recommended due to the overlap of symptoms. Even in patients with all clinical features, scoring high on having probable GAS, only 35% to 50% had confirmed GAS, particularly in children.[2-5] For this reason, it is recommended to perform rapid antigen detection test (RADT) or throat culture when GAS is suspected. Testing is not recommended for patients with overt viral features.

3. **Explanation:** The correct answer is A. GAS diagnostic testing is not indicated for children <3 years old due to unlikelihood of GAS being responsible for pharyngitis in that population. However, testing may be warranted if the child has contact with other children who have a GAS infection. GAS is responsible for 20% to 30% of sore throat visits in children, most commonly in children age 5 to 15 years of age during the cold months of winter to early spring. It is less common in adults, being responsible for 5% to 15% of acute pharyngitis cases.[6,7] Diagnostic testing by rapid antigen detection test (RADT) via throat swab is highly specific (about 95%) and is available as a CLIA-waived test that can be utilized in pharmacies and prescriber offices. RADT has a primary advantage over throat culture in that treatment, if indicated, is not delayed. However, due to lower sensitivity of the RADT (70% to 90%) it may be reasonable to confirm a negative RADT with throat culture in children.[8,9]

4. **Explanation:** The correct answer is B. Due to the patient's amoxicillin allergy with anaphylaxis, cephalosporins are not recommended for this patient. If her allergy was not anaphylactic, cephalosporins (cephalexin and cefadroxil) can serve as alternative agents. The treatment of choice for GAS pharyngitis includes penicillin V, penicillin G IM (the only injectable option, at a single dose, which is helpful for adherence), or amoxicillin, in patients who are not allergic to penicillins. While clindamycin, azithromycin, and clarithromycin are all reasonable alternatives, the general resistance to clindamycin is about 1% and resistance to the macrolides is about 5% to 8%.[1] Depending on local resistance rates, clindamycin may be preferred in this patient. For pediatrics, clindamycin is dosed 7 mg/kg/dose three times daily, at a maximum of 300 mg/dose. Based on the patient's weight of 65 lb or 29.55 kg, she requires 207 mg/dose. Azithromycin is dosed at 12 mg/kg once (maximum dose of 500 mg) followed by 6 mg/kg (maximum dose of 250 mg) for the next four days. Clarithromycin is dosed at 7.5 mg/kg/dose (maximum dose of 250 mg) twice daily for 10 days. Note that treatment duration for all oral regimens is 10 days, except azithromycin.

5. **Explanation:** The correct answer is D. Clindamycin solution should be stored at room temperature. Common side

effects include rash or diarrhea. However, these side effects could also be indicators of more rare but severe adverse effects, such as erythema multiforme, exfoliative dermatitis, Stevens–Johnson syndrome or *Clostridioides difficile* infection. Adherence is important not only for adults, but also for children. As pediatric medications are available in oral liquid dosage form, taste is a factor to consider. Taste tests have shown that clindamycin is among the most unpalatable of the liquid antimicrobials. Of the three viable antibiotics for this patient, azithromycin is the most palatable.[10]

6. **Explanation:** The correct answer is C. Adjunctive therapy with acetaminophen or a nonsteroidal anti-inflammatory drug (NSAID) is reasonable to manage the fever and pain associated with GAS pharyngitis. It is not, however, recommended to use aspirin in children due to the risk of Reye's syndrome, or corticosteroids due to potential for adverse effects and minimal efficacy in pain reduction.[1] Acetaminophen for this patient using the over-the-counter product, manufacturer dosing table, and supplied dosing cup is 400 mg (12.5 mL) given every 4 to 6 hours. It should not be given more than five times a day.[11] Alternatively, the weight-based dosing is 10 to 15 mg/kg/dose using the 160 mg/5 mL oral suspension. Additionally, JT should discontinue her herbal remedy, as it has not been effective thus far, and the evidence regarding safety and efficacy is insufficient.[12]

7. **Explanation:** The correct answer is C. While medication noncompliance and new GAS infections from community contacts can occur, given the multiple infections while being GAS-positive as well as symptoms likely indicative of a viral infection, JT may be a chronic pharyngeal GAS carrier (hence the positive GAS RADT) experiencing recurrent infections of viral origin. Patients identified as being a chronic pharyngeal GAS carrier generally do not require antimicrobial therapy as they are unlikely to transmit GAS pharyngitis to other close contacts and have little risk of developing further complications. At times, it may be difficult to differentiate new GAS infection from new viral infections while being a GAS carrier, so signs and symptoms, local epidemiology, age, and season should be considered.[1]

8. **Explanation:** The correct answer is B. It is not recommended to perform a tonsillectomy for prophylaxis of GAS pharyngitis. Tonsillectomy may be considered in rare cases in which there are unexplainable, persistent, recurrent episodes of GAS pharyngitis, though long-term benefits are unknown.[1]

REFERENCES

1. Shulman ST, Bisno AL, Clegg HW, et al. Clinical practice guideline for the diagnosis and management of group a streptococcal pharyngitis: 2012 update by the Infectious Diseases Society of America. *Clin Infect Dis.* 2012;55(10):e86-e102.
2. Bisno AL, Gerber MA, Gwaltney JM, et al. Practice guidelines for the diagnosis and management of group a streptococcal pharyngitis. *Clin Infect Dis.* 2002;35(2):113-125.
3. Choby BA. Diagnosis and treatment of streptococcal pharyngitis. *Am Fam Physician.* 2009;79(5):383-390.
4. McIsaac WJ, Keller JD, Aufricht P, Vajanka A, Low DE. Empirical validation of guidelines for the management of pharyngitis in children and adults. *JAMA.* 2004;291:587-595.
5. Kaplan EL, Top FH Jr, Dudding BA, Wannamaker LW. Diagnosis of streptococcal pharyngitis: differentiation of active infection from the carrier state in the symptomatic child. *J Infect Dis.* 1971;123:490-501.
6. Bisno AL. Acute pharyngitis: etiology and diagnosis. *Pediatrics.* 1996;97:949-954.
7. Ebell MH, Smith MA, Barry HC, Ives K, Carey M. The rational clinical examination. Does this patient have strep throat? *JAMA.* 2000;284:2908-2912.
8. Gerber MA, Shulman ST. Rapid diagnosis of pharyngitis caused by group A streptococci. *Clin Microbiol Rev.* 2004;17:571-580.
9. Tanz RR, Gerber MA, Kabat W, Rippe J, Seshadri R, Shulman ST. Performance of a rapid antigen-detection test and throat culture in community pediatric offices: implications for management of pharyngitis. *Pediatrics.* 2009;123:437-444.
10. Gee SC, Hagemann TM. Palatability of liquid anti-infectives: clinican and student perceptions and practice outcomes. *J Pediatr Pharmacol Ther.* 2007;12:216-223.
11. Children's Tylenol® [drug facts]. Johnson & Johnson Consumer Inc., Mcneil Consumer Healthcare Division; 2018.
12. Nin Jiom Pei Pa Koa [drug facts]. Nin Jiom Medicine Manufactory (HK) Ltd; 2011.

5 Community-Acquired Pneumonia

Sean N. Avedissian   Marc H. Scheetz

PATIENT PRESENTATION

Chief Complaint

"I have been coughing, have chest pain, and cannot breathe for about 2 days now."

History of Present Illness

WA is a 40-year-old Caucasian male who presents to the emergency department with a fever, cough, chest pain (worsening when breathing or coughing), and shortness of breath. Normally, he has a fairly active lifestyle as he trains for marathons. He has not traveled outside the United States recently. He states he has "been taking cough medicine at night" for the past 4 days to help him sleep, but it has not been getting better. Also, he reports that he has been waking up at night due to heavy sweating. He states all his symptoms have gotten worse in the last 2 days. After being assessed in the ED, WA is admitted to the medicine unit for further workup.

Past Medical History

Diabetes: Type 1

Surgical History

N/A

Family History

Father has diabetes: Type 1, history of heart attack; mother has hypertension.

Social History

Married with no kids. Denies smoking and drinks alcohol occasionally (weekends, social events)

Allergies

NKDA

Home Medications

Insulin (bolus/basal: ~35 units total daily)
Aspirin 81 mg PO daily (cardiovascular protection)
Atorvastatin 20 mg PO daily (cardiovascular protection)

Physical Examination

▸ **Vital Signs**

Temp 100.8°F, HR 110 bpm, RR 30, BP 125/75 mm Hg, p02 93%, Ht 5′9″, Wt 70 kg

▸ **General**

Slightly lethargic, mild—moderate distress

▸ **HEENT**

Normocephalic, atraumatic, PERRLA, EOMI, normal mucus membranes and conjunctiva, adequate dentition

▸ **Pulmonary**

Diminished breath sounds and crackles (rales) bilaterally

▸ **Cardiovascular**

NSR, no m/r/g

▸ **Abdomen**

Soft, non-distended, non-tender, bowel sounds hyperactive

▸ **Neurology**

Lethargic, oriented to place and person, (–) Brudzinski's sign, (–) Kernig's sign

▸ **Extremities**

No significant findings

▶ **Vaccines**

States he cannot remember all of them. He says he received all his age-related vaccines when younger. Has not received his flu-shot this year as he always forgets to receive it.

Laboratory Findings

Na = 148, mEq/L	Hgb = 14 g/dL	Ca = 8.5 mg/dL
K = 4.3 mEq/L	Hct = 38%	Mg = 2.3 mg/dL
CL = 115 mEq/L	Plt = 300 × 10³/mm³	Phos = 4 mg/dL
CO₂ = 28 mEq/L	WBC = 18 × 10³ mm³	AST = 21 IU/L
BUN = 20 mg/dL	Trop <0.01 ng/mL	ALT = 35 IU/L
SCr = 0.9 mg/dL	CK = 1.8 ng/mL	T-Bili = 0.5 mg/dL
Glu = 140 mg/dL	BNP = 30 pg/mL	Alk Phos = 60 IU/L
Procalcitonin = 0.8 mcg/L		

▶ **Chest X-ray**

Consolidation, pleural effusions present

▶ **Blood Cultures**

NGTD

▶ **Sputum Culture (high-quality)**

Pending

▶ **NARES MRSA PCR**

Negative

▶ **Urine Antigen Test**

Legionella (negative), *Pneumococcal* (negative)

▶ **Respiratory Pathogen Panel (RPP)**

Negative

QUESTIONS

1. What is WA's CURB-65 score?
   A. 1
   B. 2
   C. 3
   D. 4

2. What findings does WA present with that will aid in the diagnosis of a patient positive for community-acquired pneumonia (CAP)?
   A. Chest X-ray findings
   B. Blood culture findings
   C. Urine antigen test findings
   D. His PMH

3. What empiric antibiotic(s) therapy would you start on WA for community-acquired pneumonia (CAP)?
   A. Azithromycin
   B. Ceftriaxone
   C. Ceftriaxone plus azithromycin
   D. Ceftriaxone plus vancomycin
   E. Piperacillin-tazobactam plus azithromycin

4. Which of the following is *not* an adverse effects of fluoroquinolones?
   A. QTc prolongation
   B. Glucose abnormalities
   C. Tendinopathy/tendon rupture
   D. Aplastic anemia

5. As per CAP guideline recommendations,[1] which of the following is not a reason to switch WA to oral antibiotic therapy?
   A. Hemodynamic stability with clinical improvement
   B. Ability to ingest medications
   C. Failing IV therapy
   D. Normally function gastrointestinal tract

6. What would be an appropriate total duration of therapy (days) of antibiotic(s) for WA if he is showing clinical improvement?
   A. 4 days
   B. 5 days
   C. 7 days
   D. 10 days

7. What vaccine(s) would you recommend (including seasonal vaccines) that WA receive (assuming he has not already received them)?
   A. Annual influenza vaccine + 23-valent pneumococcal polysaccharide vaccine (PPSV23)
   B. 23-valent pneumococcal polysaccharide vaccine (PPSV23)
   C. 13-valent pneumococcal conjugate vaccine (PCV13)
   D. Annual influenza vaccine + 13-valent pneumococcal conjugate vaccine (PCV13)

ANSWERS

1. **Explanation:** The correct answer is B, i.e., 2. The CURB-65 is one example of a severity-of-illness index that can be useful for assessing the mortality risk and need for hospitalization in patients with community acquired pneumonia. For WA, his CURB-65 score is equal to 2 because he has an RR ≥30 breaths/min and an urea greater than 19 mg/dL.
   CURB-65 Criteria:[1]
   Confusion, new onset
   Urea greater than 19 mg/dL
   Respiratory rate of 30 breaths/min or more

Blood pressure of 90 mm Hg or less systolic or diastolic of 60 mm Hg or less

Age **65** years or older

Each criterion counts as 1 point; score of 0 = 0.7% mortality risk, 1 = 2.1%, 2 = 9.2%, 3 = 14.5%, 4 = 40%. Consider hospitalization if the CURB-65 score is 2 or more.

2. **Explanation:** The correct answer is A, chest X-ray findings. The consolidation with pleural effusions is consistent with CAP. As the rest of the choices can provide essential information in patients with CAP, they are not clinically significant in WA's presentation.

3. **Explanation:** The correct answer is C, ceftriaxone plus azithromycin. Given that the sputum Gram stain is still pending, ceftriaxone would cover the potential typical pathogens (i.e., *S. pneumoniae* vs. *H. influenzae*) for CAP. CAP empiric treatment also includes coverage of atypical organisms (*C. pneumoniae*, *M. pneumoniae*, *L. pneumophila*). Thus, a macrolide such as azithromycin is recommended for added coverage. However, a macrolide should not be used as monotherapy due to high *S. pneumoniae* resistance rates, especially in patients with comorbidities such as type 1 DM. The current 2007 guideline lists levofloxacin (fluoroquinolone) as an option (but this was not a possible answer listed for this question). However, given resistance development, adverse effects, and strengthened FDA warnings, the usage of fluoroquinolones should be reserved for patients who have no alternative treatment options. It is unclear how the new CAP guidelines (currently in development) will classify fluoroquinolone treatment for CAP. While WA's *Legionella* antigen is negative, you cannot rule out other atypical pathogens at this time given cultures are still pending, and most atypical bacteria are not detectable on Gram stain or cultivatable on standard bacteriologic media. Further, adding vancomycin is not recommended given the patient does not present with MRSA-specific risk factors/MRSA-consistent clinical presentation. WA's MRSA PCR is also negative, which has a high negative predictive value for MRSA PNA. Finally, piperacillin-tazobactam would only be needed if the patient presented with gram-negative risk factors.[3] As per guideline recommendations, it is also important to consider the floor the patient is admitted to when deciding on empiric treatment because recommendations will differ if treating outpatient vs. inpatient (non-ICU) vs. inpatient (ICU). Please refer to guidelines for more information.

Summary of IDSA Guidelines	
MRSA-specific PNA risk factors • Dialysis (PD or HD)/end-stage renal disease • Injection drug abuse • Prior influenza • Prior antibiotic therapy (especially with fluoroquinolones) • Prior MRSA colonization or infection • Necrotizing or cavitary PNA	Consider adding vancomycin or linezolid for MRSA coverage.
Gram-negative PNA risk factors • Severe COPD • Smoking • Alcoholism • Aspiration • Recent use of antibiotics (within 3 months)	Consider piperacillin-tazobactam or cefepime + azithromycin.
MRSA-consistent clinical presentation of PNA suspicious with gene for Panton-Valentine leukocidin (necrotizing PNA) • Shock • Respiratory failure • Formation of abscesses and empyema	Patients who present with these symptoms are at high risk for toxin-producing MRSA strains. Addition of clindamycin or use of linezolid may be considered for their potential toxin inhibitory effects.[2,3]

Source: Data from references 1, 2, and 3.

4. **Explanation:** The correct answer is D, aplastic anemia. Options A through C are very serious and important adverse drug effects to be able to identify for fluoroquinolones. Option B is especially significant for WA given his type 1 DM diagnosis. Option D is less specific for fluoroquinolones and would be more commonly associated with an antibiotic such as chloramphenicol.

5. **Explanation:** The correct answer is C, failing IV therapy. All other choices are criteria provided by the CAP

guidelines as reasons to consider switching a patient to oral therapy. If a patient is failing IV therapy, a discussion about if the antibiotic is appropriately covering the potential pathogen(s) should happen with the health care team. The goal is to discharge patients as soon as they are clinically stable, have no other active medical problems, and have a safe environment for continued care. Further, it is not necessary to keep the patient admitted while receiving oral therapy if patient is clinical stable.

6. **Explanation:** The best answer would be B, 5 days. If the patient is showing clinical improvement, which is specified in the question, a shorter total days of therapy is recommended. Historically, patients received 7 to 10 days of treatment for CAP. The 2007 IDSA CAP guidelines[1] recommend that patients receive at least 5 days, depending on clinical stability. Clinical stability includes temperature ≤37.8°C, heart rate ≤100 beats/min, respiratory rate ≤24 breaths/min, systolic blood pressure ≥90 mm Hg, arterial oxygen saturation ≥90%, and ability to maintain oral intake and normal mental status. Further, patients should be afebrile for 48 to 7 hours with no more than 1 CAP-associated sign of clinical instability. More recently, an RCT[4] evaluated decision making for the duration of therapy in patients with CAP and found that 5 days of therapy was safe in the studied population when patients met criteria for clinical stability. There are many benefits to shorter duration for CAP treatment, which include decreased risk of developing colonization with penicillin-resistant *S. pneumoniae* when using β-lactams, decreased risk of adverse drug effects, including *C. difficile* infection, and improved adherence and decreased cost.

7. **Explanation:** The correct answer would be A. Given that WA is diabetic (Type 1), the influenza vaccine (received annually) and the PPSV23 vaccine are recommended for those ≥19 years.[5] As it is unclear if WA received his PCV13 vaccine in the past, current ACIP guidelines only recommend PPSV23. Annual vaccination remains the primary tool for influenza prevention; everyone at least 6 months of age should receive an annual vaccination. Effectiveness of the influenza vaccination varies year by year, depending on how well matched the strains are to the vaccine components. The complete vaccination recommendation table can be found in reference 5.

REFERENCES

1. Mandell LA, Wunderink RG, Anzueto A, et al.; Infectious Diseases Society of America, American Thoracic Society. Infectious Diseases Society of America/American Thoracic Society consensus guidelines on the management of community-acquired pneumonia in adults. *Clin Infect Dis.* 2007;44(suppl 2):S27-S72.
2. Gillet Y, Vanhems P, Lina G, et al. Factors predicting mortality in necrotizing community-acquired pneumonia caused by *Staphylococcus aureus* containing Panton-Valentine leukocidin. *Clin Infect Dis.* 2007;45:315-321.
3. Bernardo K, Pakulat N, Fleer S, et al. Subinhibitory concentrations of linezolid reduce *Staphylococcus aureus* virulence factor expression. *Antimicrob Agents Chemother.* 2004;48:546-555.
4. Uranga A, Espana PP, Bilbao A, et al. Duration of antibiotic treatment in community-acquired pneumonia: A multicenter randomized clinical trial. *JAMA Intern Med.* 2016;176:1257-1265.
5. Bennett NM, Whitney CG, Moore M, Pilishvili T, Dooling KL. Use of 13-valent pneumococcal conjugate vaccine and 23-valent pneumococcal polysaccharide vaccine for adults with immunocompromising conditions: Recommendations of the Advisory Committee on Immunization Practices (ACIP) (Reprinted from MMWR vol 40, pg 816, 2012). *J Am Med Assoc.* 2013;309:334-336.

6 Hospital-Acquired and Ventilator-Associated Pneumonia

Stephanie E. Giancola   Elizabeth B. Hirsch

PATIENT PRESENTATION

History of Present Illness

RW is a 67-year-old man who was transported to Acute Care Medical Center (ACMC) after being struck by a car while crossing First Avenue on foot. He has been hospitalized at ACMC for 6 days and is in the trauma ICU due to several fractures sustained in the motor vehicle accident. The patient has been intubated and on mechanical ventilation since admission 6 days ago. During ICU rounds the next morning, the nurse notes he has had increased, yellow/green secretions overnight.

Past Medical History

Hypertension
Type 2 diabetes mellitus

Family History

Mother died from a myocardial infarction at age 84. Father is still living in nursing home, has past history of prostate cancer.

Social History

The patient is an engineering professor at the State University. He is married and lives at home with his wife. He has 2 college-age kids attending college outside of the metro area. As per his wife, he has not traveled outside the local area for the past 6 months, but he traveled to Germany about a year ago. There are no pets in the home. He drinks 2 to 3 beers per week.

Current Medications

Sodium chloride 0.9% (NS) @ 150 mL/hr
Heparin 5000 units subcutaneously q8 h
Insulin infusion titrated to maintain BG 80-110
Fentanyl intravenous infusion at 25 mcg/hr
Dexmedetomidine intravenous infusion titrated to RASS 0 to –2

Allergies

NKDA

Home Medications

Lisinopril/hydrochlorothiazide 20/12.5 mg PO daily
Metformin 1000 mg PO BID
No recent antibiotic use within the past 6 months

▶ Vital Signs

Temp 101.3°F, BP 110/72 mm Hg, HR 80 to 90 bpm, RR 21 breaths per minute, SpO_2 92% on mechanical ventilation
Ht 6'1" Wt 98 kg

▶ General

Intubated, no acute distress

▶ HEENT

Normocephalic, atraumatic, EOMI, PERRLA, MMM, no adenopathy

▶ Cardiovascular

No m/r/g, normal S1/S2

▶ Pulmonary

Crackles in the right posterior base with dullness: left lung clear

▶ Abdomen

Soft, non-tender, non-distended with positive bowel sounds

▶ Genitourinary

Urinary (Foley) catheter is in place

▶ Extremities

LLE in ace wrap and post-op bandages, LUE in post-op bandages

▶ *Neurology*

Alert and oriented × 2 upon admission (person and place, not date)

Laboratory Findings

WBC 12.2 ×10³/μL (8% bands), platelets 156 ×10³/μL, AST/ALT 54/32 units/L, SCr 1.5 mg/dL, lactate 1.1 mmol/L, albumin 2.2 g/dL, INR 1.2, blood glucose (3 most recent q4h accuchecks = 110, 80, 90 mg/dL) and all other laboratory values are WNL

▶ *Pertinent Ventilator Settings*

FiO_2: 60% (increased from 40% yesterday)
PEEP: 8 cm H_2O (increased from 5 cm H_2O yesterday)

QUESTIONS

1. What signs/symptoms does RW have that are consistent with the presentation of pneumonia?
   A. Increased sputum production
   B. Increased ventilator settings (FiO_2 and PEEP)
   C. Crackles on auscultation
   D. A and B
   E. A, B, and C

2. Which diagnostic procedures would be indicated in RW at the current time?
   A. Chest X-ray
   B. Endotracheal culture
   C. Bronchoalveolar lavage (BAL)
   D. A and B
   E. A and C

3. A portable CXR is obtained on day 6, which shows a new infiltrate in the right lower lobe. Which infectious syndrome would be highest on the differential diagnosis?
   A. Community-acquired pneumonia (CAP)
   B. Hospital-acquired pneumonia (HAP)
   C. Ventilator-associated pneumonia (VAP)
   D. Ventilator-associated tracheobronchitis (VAT)

4. The hospital's antibiogram shows the following susceptibility data.

Organism	Drug	Percent susceptible
Staphylococcus aureus	Oxacillin	68%
	Vancomycin	100%
Pseudomonas aeruginosa	Piperacillin-tazobactam	84%
	Cefepime	90%
	Meropenem	93%
	Ciprofloxacin	78%
	Tobramycin	91%

Which antibiotic regimen would be most correct for empiric treatment in RW?
   A. Cefepime + tobramycin + vancomycin
   B. Ciprofloxacin + ceftriaxone + vancomycin
   C. Piperacillin-tazobactam + vancomycin
   D. Meropenem + levofloxacin
   E. Meropenem

5. If the patient was not ventilated, what empiric antibiotic regimen would be recommended?
   A. Cefepime + tobramycin + vancomycin
   B. Cefepime + vancomycin
   C. Piperacillin-tazobactam + levofloxacin + linezolid
   D. Meropenem + levofloxacin
   E. Meropenem

6. Regardless of your recommendation above, the patient is started on piperacillin-tazobactam 4.5 g IV q6h plus levofloxacin 750 mg IV daily plus vancomycin 1500 mg IV q24h, and is clinically improving on this regimen with low risk for mortality (<15%). Cultures return 48 hours later and reveal the following:

   Blood cultures: negative
   Endotracheal aspirate culture: positive for 3+ *Pseudomonas aeruginosa*

Amikacin	S
Cefepime	S
Ceftazidime	S
Ciprofloxacin	R
Meropenem	S
Piperacillin-tazobactam	S
Tobramycin	S

   R = resistant; S = susceptible.

   Which of the following definitive antibiotic regimens should now be recommended for RW?
   A. Discontinue piperacillin-tazobactam, levofloxacin, and vancomycin; start meropenem monotherapy
   B. Discontinue levofloxacin and vancomycin; continue piperacillin-tazobactam and add tobramycin
   C. Discontinue piperacillin-tazobactam, levofloxacin, and vancomycin; start tobramycin monotherapy
   D. Discontinue piperacillin-tazobactam, levofloxacin, and vancomycin; start cefepime monotherapy

7. What total duration of antibiotic therapy would be recommended for RW's VAP?
   A. 5 days
   B. 7 days
   C. 10 days
   D. 14 days

ANSWERS

1. **Explanation:** The correct answer is E (i.e., all of the above). Increased sputum production, increased ventilator settings

(FiO$_2$ and PEEP), and crackles on auscultation are all signs or symptoms of pneumonia. Additional signs/symptoms that are consistent with pneumonia include fever, chest pain, cough, dyspnea, leukocytosis, and decreased oxygen saturation.

2. **Explanation:** The correct answer is D. A chest X-ray would be essential for the diagnosis of pneumonia. Since the patient is hospitalized in the ICU, sputum cultures, blood cultures, urinary antigen tests (UAT; for *Streptococcus pneumoniae* and *Legionella* spp.) could all be ordered. Since the patient is still intubated, an endotracheal culture is now recommended as per the most recent 2016 Infectious Diseases Society of America (IDSA) and American Thoracic Society (ATS) guidelines.[1] Bronchoscopy would not be indicated at this time since there is no real reason to do this invasive procedure if no sputum cultures have been done yet. Rationale for this recommendation is based on the lack of evidence that invasive (i.e., bronchoscopy) microbiological sampling with quantitative cultures improves clinical outcomes as compared to noninvasive sampling.[1] Noninvasive sampling can also be done rapidly, with fewer complications and resources.

3. **Explanation:** The correct answer is C. CAP is defined as pneumonia that developed in the community with symptoms beginning prior to presentation and up to 48 hours after hospital admission (rules out option A). HAP is defined as pneumonia that occurs 48 hours or more after admission in non-ventilated patients (rules out option B). VAT is defined as fever with no other recognizable cause, with new or increased sputum production, positive endotracheal aspirate culture, and no radiographic evidence of nosocomial pneumonia (rules out option D). VAP is defined as pneumonia that arises more than 48 hours after endotracheal intubation. RW has been intubated for 6 days, has signs/symptoms of pneumonia, and has radiographic evidence of pneumonia; therefore, answer C is correct.

4. **Explanation:** The correct answer is A. In patients with suspected VAP, the empiric antibiotic regimen should include coverage for *Staphylococcus aureus, Pseudomonas aeruginosa,* and other gram-negative bacilli. The choice of antibiotics to cover these organisms depends on risk factors for resistance.[1] An antibiotic active against methicillin-resistant *S. aureus* (MRSA) is indicated if the patient has one of the risk factors listed in the Table 6.1.[1] If no risk factors are present, then an agent active against methicillin-susceptible *S. aureus* (MSSA) is recommended. Two antibiotics from different antibiotic classes active against *P. aeruginosa* are recommended if the patient has one of the risk factors listed in Table 6.1. If no risk factors are present, then one antibiotic active against *P. aeruginosa* is recommended. RW has been hospitalized for 6 days; therefore, an agent active against MRSA (rules out options D and E) and 2 antipseudomonal agents (rules out options B and C) are indicated. Answer A is the only option that includes 2 antipseudomonal agents and an agent active against MRSA. Of note, before starting any antibiotic regimen,

the patient's allergies should be verified. In this case, the patient has no known drug allergies.

TABLE 6.1. Risk Factors for Resistance for VAP

MDR VAP (MRSA and MDR *P. aeruginosa*)	MRSA VAP	MDR *Pseudomonas* VAP
• Prior IV antibiotic use within 90 days • Septic shock at the time of VAP • ARDS preceding VAP • Five or more days of hospitalization prior to the occurrence of VAP • Acute renal replacement therapy prior to VAP onset	• Patients in units where >10–20% of *S. aureus* isolates are methicillin resistant • Patients in units where the prevalence of MRSA is not known	• Patients in units where >10% of gram-negative isolates are resistant to an agent being considered for monotherapy • Patients in units where local antimicrobial susceptibility rates are unknown • Bronchiectasis • Cystic fibrosis

5. **Explanation:** The correct answer is B. If the patient was not ventilated, the patient's pneumonia would be classified as HAP. Similar to treatment of VAP, the choice of empiric antibiotics to treat HAP depends on risk factors for resistance. However, risk factors for resistance in HAP are slightly different from those in VAP, as shown in Table 6.2 below.[1] An antibiotic active against MRSA and 2 antibiotics active against *Pseudomonas* are indicated if a risk factor

TABLE 6.2. Risk Factors for Resistance for HAP

MDR HAP (MRSA and MDR *P. aeruginosa*)	MRSA HAP	MDR *Pseudomonas* HAP
• Prior IV antibiotic use within 90 days • Septic shock • Need for ventilator support due to HAP	• Patients in units where >20% of *S. aureus* isolates are methicillin resistant • Patients in units where the prevalence of MRSA is not known	• Bronchiectasis • Cystic fibrosis

for resistance is present. RW is hospitalized in a unit where >20% of *S. aureus* isolate are resistant to oxacillin. No other risk factors for resistance are present. Therefore, an agent active against MRSA (rules out options D and E) plus one agent active against *P. aeruginosa* (rules out options A and C) are indicated for RW. Answer B is the only option that includes one antipseudomonal agent and an agent active against MRSA.

6. **Explanation:** The correct answer is D. When HAP or VAP is due to *P. aeruginosa,* monotherapy with an antibiotic to which the isolate is susceptible is recommended rather than combination therapy unless the patient is in septic shock or is at high risk for mortality, defined as >25% (rules out option B).[2] This patient has a low risk of mortality (stated as <15% in question) and has a normal MAP (85 mm Hg) and normal lactate level and is thus not in septic shock. Aminoglycosides are not recommended as monotherapy due to their poor lung penetration and lack of studies evaluating the effects of aminoglycoside monotherapy for VAP or HAP (rules out option C). Both meropenem and cefepime will effectively treat this patient's infection. To choose between these two options, antimicrobial stewardship principles should be considered. When recommending definitive therapy, de-escalating therapy to the narrowest spectrum agent that will effectively treat the infection is generally recommended. In this case, cefepime is narrower in spectrum of activity than carbapenems and choosing meropenem carries higher risk for the development of carbapenem resistance, which has limited treatment options (rules out A). Therefore, answer D is correct.

7. **Explanation:** The correct answer is B. Several studies have assessed the optimal duration of therapy for VAP by comparing short durations (7–8 days) to longer durations (10–15 days).[3-5] Most data showed no difference in mortality, clinical cure/treatment failure, or hospital length of stay.

However, older data have shown conflicting results and increased frequency of recurrent pneumonia in patients with VAP receiving short-course therapy due to non-lactose fermenting gram-negative bacilli, including *Pseudomonas* spp. Therefore, the authors of the 2016 guidelines by the IDSA and ATS performed their own meta-analysis to answer this question.[1] They found no difference in mortality, clinical cure, or recurrent pneumonia, including in the subgroup of patients with non-lactose fermenting gram-negative bacilli. Therefore, the shorter duration of 7 days of therapy is recommended, making answer B correct.

REFERENCES

1. Kalil AC, Metersky ML, Klompas M, et al. Management of adults with hospital-acquired and ventilator-associated pneumonia: 2016 clinical practice guidelines by the Infectious Diseases Society of America and the American Thoracic Society. *Clin Infect Dis.* 2016;63(5):e61-e111.

2. Kumar A, Safdar N, Kethireddy S, Chateau D. A survival benefit of combination antibiotic therapy for serious infections associated with sepsis and septic shock is contingent only on the risk of death: a meta-analytic/meta-regression study. *Crit Care Med.* 2010;38(8):1651-1664.

3. Chastre J, Wolff M, Fagon JY, et al. Comparison of 8 vs 15 days of antibiotic therapy for ventilator-associated pneumonia in adults: a randomized trial. *JAMA.* 2003;290(19):2588-2598.

4. Capellier G, Mockly H, Charpentier C, et al. Early-onset ventilator-associated pneumonia in adults randomized clinical trial: comparison of 8 versus 15 days of antibiotic treatment. *PLoS One.* 2012;7(8):e41290.

5. Pugh R, Grant C, Cooke RP, Dempsey G. Short-course versus prolonged-course antibiotic therapy for hospital-acquired pneumonia in critically ill adults. *Cochrane Database Syst Rev.* 2015(8):CD007577.

7 Cystitis

Kristy M. Shaeer

PATIENT PRESENTATION

Chief Complaint

"I have painful and frequent urination."

History of Present Illness

VZ is a 19-year-old Hispanic female who presents to the urgent care walk-in clinic with dysuria and polyuria for 3 days duration.

Past Medical History

Seasonal allergies

Surgical History

None

Family History

Mother has HTN; father has HTN, type 2 diabetes mellitus, and dyslipidemia

Social History

Currently attending college as a sophomore. Smokes tobacco and marijuana cigarettes socially on weekends for the past 2 years; drinks alcohol (beer and wine) socially on weekends for the past year. Sexually active with her boyfriend of 8 months; uses condoms

Allergies

Sulfas-rash and blisters

Home Medications

Ethinyl estradiol/etonogestrel 0.015 mg/0.12 mg unwrap and insert one ring intravaginally and remove every 21 days then repeat 7 days later
Cetirizine 10 mg PO daily PRN seasonal allergies
Triamcinolone acetonide 55 mcg/spray 1–2 sprays EN PRN seasonal allergies
Phenazopyridine hydrochloride 200 mg PO TID after meals

Physical Examination

▶ Vital Signs

Temp 98.4°F, P 62, RR 10 breaths per minute, BP 112/82 mm Hg, pO_2 98%, Ht 5′6″, Wt 52.3 kg

▶ General

Thin, well-nourished female, lying in bed, NAD, AAO × 3

▶ HEENT

EOMI, PERRLA, normocephalic, no pharyngeal exudate. Neck, supple. Thyroid palpable, no nodules. No lymphadenopathy

▶ Pulmonary

CTAB without wheezing or crackles

▶ Cardiovascular

NSR, no m/r/g

▶ Abdomen

Soft, non-distended, non-tender, positive bowel sounds hyperactive, no rebound or guarding

▶ Genitourinary

Normal female genitalia, complaints of dysuria, denies hematuria. No malodorous discharge noted from vagina

▶ Neurology

PERRLA, no focal deficits noted

▶ Extremities

Edema present in lower extremity bilaterally. Pedal pulses palpable

▶ Back

No tenderness to palpation on lower lumbar region

Laboratory Findings

Dipstick Urinalysis:

Macroscopic: urine midstream, clean catch. Yellow, cloudy, large leukocytes, positive nitrites, urine pH = 8, urine hemoglobin, protein, glucose, ketones, and bilirubin negative, specific gravity = 1.012

Microscopic: WBCs >100, RBCs 0, squamous epithelial cells 0, few WBC clumps

▶ Urine Gram Stain

Many gram-negative rods

QUESTIONS

1. Which of the following symptom(s) is/are suggestive of cystitis? Select all that apply.
   A. Flank pain
   B. Dysuria
   C. Polyuria
   D. Fever

2. Which components of VZ's urinalysis are often suggestive of a urinary tract infection (UTI)? Select all that apply.
   A. Specific gravity
   B. Leukocyte esterase
   C. pH
   D. Nitrites
   E. RBCs

3. Which empiric agent would be most appropriate for VZ's cystitis?
   A. Amoxicillin
   B. Levofloxacin
   C. Aztreonam
   D. Trimethoprim-sulfamethoxazole
   E. Nitrofurantoin

4. How many day(s) would be the most appropriate duration of therapy?
   A. 1
   B. 3
   C. 5
   D. 7
   E. 10

5. The urinalysis and culture is suggestive of which of the following organisms?

   Urine culture: gram-negative lactose-fermenting rods
   A. *Escherichia coli*
   B. *Acinetobacter baumanii*
   C. *Enterococcocus faecalis*
   D. *Staphylococcus aureus*
   E. *Stenotrophomonas maltophilia*

6. Although unnecessary, the provider sent the urine sample for culture and the following susceptibilities to various agents. Which of the agents below is the most appropriate option for treatment?

Susceptibility Report	
Amikacin	≤2
Amoxicillin/Clavulanate	≤2
Ampicillin	≤2
Ampicillin/Sulbactam	≤2
Aztreonam	≤1
Cefazolin	≤4
Cefepime	≤1
Cefotaxime	≤1
Cefotetan	≤4
Cefoxitin	≤4
Cefpodoxime	≤0.25
Ceftazidime	≤1
Ceftriaxone	≤1
Cefuroxime axetil	4
Cefuroxime-Sodium	4
Ciprofloxacin	≤0.25
Ertapenem	≤0.5
Gentamicin	≤1
Imipenem	≤0.25
Levofloxacin	≤0.12
Meropenem	≤0.25
Nitrofurantoin	≤16
Piperacillin/Tazobactam	≤4
Tetracycline	≤1
Tobramycin	≤1
Trimethoprim/Sulfamethoxazole	≤20

   A. Amoxicillin
   B. Nitrofurantoin
   C. Cefepime
   D. Cephalexin
   E. Trimethoprim-sulfamethoxazole

7. VZ has been taking phenazopyridine for the last 24 hours. Which of the following are appropriate counseling points about this over-the-counter medication? Select all that apply.
   A. Avoid using for more than 48 hours longer with a total duration of 72 hours
   B. Avoid using for more than 24 hours longer with a total duration of 48 hours
   C. Produces a red to orange discoloration of the urine and sclera leading to staining of clothing and contact lenses
   D. Produces a bluish green discoloration of the urine and sclera leading to staining of clothing and contact lenses
   E. Not intended to treat a UTI and will help minimize dysuria

ANSWERS

1. **Explanation:** Correct answers are B and C. Dysuria, polyuria, urgency, and suprapubic pain are symptoms of cystitis. Flank pain and fever are commonly seen in pyelonephritis.[1] Uncomplicated cystitis is defined as urgency, frequency, dysuria, suprapubic pain/tenderness, in an otherwise healthy, nonpregnant woman who lacks fever, flank pain, tenderness, and vaginal discharge.[1,2]

2. **Explanation:** Correct answers are B, C, and D.[3] Leukocyte esterase is an enzyme that is produced by neutrophils and may indicate pyuria associated with a UTI. Urinary pH can range from 4.5 to 8 but normally is slightly acidic

(eg, 5.5–6.5) because of metabolic activity. Alkaline urine can be seen in patients with a UTI.[2,3] Nitrites are not typically found in urine and result when bacteria reduce urinary nitrates to nitrites. Not all bacteria are capable of this conversion, thus a positive nitrite is helpful but a negative test does not exclude a UTI. Organisms from the Enterobacteriaceae family (eg, *E. coli*, *Klebsiella* spp., *Enterobacter* spp., *Proteus* spp.) and *Staphylococcus* spp., and *Pseudomonas* spp. reduce nitrate to nitrite in the urine. Urinary specific gravity correlates with urine osmolality and gives important insight into a patient's hydration status. It also reflects the concentrating ability of the kidneys. Normal range is typically 1.003 to 1.030. RBCs can be detected in a variety of conditions and is not specific to diagnosis of a UTI.

3. **Explanation:** Correct answer is E.[1] Nitrofurantoin is an appropriate first-line empirical agent for treatment of cystitis. Nitrofurantoin has many attractive characteristics that make it a first-line option such as its low cost, availability as an oral agent, tolerability, minimal resistance to common urinary pathogens, and less likely to cause collateral damage (eg, more focused spectrum of activity and less adverse effects on normal flora). Amoxicillin and ampicillin should not be used for empirical treatment given the relatively poor efficacy and high rates of resistance. Levofloxacin is a broad-spectrum agent that is second-line and typically unnecessary as empiric therapy for a healthy young woman with cystitis. Fluoroquinolones are second-line (eg, alternative) agents given rising rates of resistance, risk of collateral damage (eg, ecological adverse effects of antimicrobial therapy), and reserved for more serious infections. Aztreonam is an intravenous agent that should be reserved for a hospitalized patient with a severe beta-lactam allergy. The patient has a sulfa allergy; therefore, trimethoprim-sulfamethoxazole should be avoided. In addition, empiric trimethoprim-sulfamethoxazole should be avoided if resistance prevalence is known to exceed 20% or if the patient used it for UTI in previous 3 months.

4. **Explanation:** Correct answer is C.[1,4–6] Nitrofurantoin is prescribed for 5 days. Trimethoprim-sulfamethoxazole can be prescribed for just 3 days to eradicate cystitis. Hooton et al. reported that after 6 weeks, women treated for cystitis had 82% ($n = 32/39$) cure with trimethoprim-sulfamethoxazole for 3 days compared with 61% ($n = 22/36$) with nitrofurantoin ($P = 0.04$).[4] Gupta et al. compared a 3-day course of trimethoprim-sulfamethoxazole with a 5-day course of nitrofurantoin in women with cystitis. The overall clinical cure rate at 30 days was 79% ($n = 117/148$) in the trimethoprim-sulfamethoxazole group and 84% among the nitrofurantoin group (nonsignificant difference of −5%, 95% confidence interval: 4–13%).[5] Fosfomycin can be given as a single dose and has comparable efficacy to other commonly used agents for cystitis (average: 93%; range: 84–95%).[1,6] A single dose of fosfomycin was compared to a 7-day course of nitrofurantoin, which demonstrated that the early clinical response rates (cure or improvement at 5–11 days after starting therapy) were not significantly different at 91%

($n = 240/263$ women) vs. 95% ($n = 232/245$ women).[6] Some beta-lactam agents can be prescribed for 5 to 7 days only if susceptibilities are known.[1] The 7- to 10-day duration is excessive and reserved for other types of UTIs.[1] Fluoroquinolones have also demonstrated equivalent cure rates for a 3 days vs. 7 days and with higher adverse effects in the longer treatment group.[1]

5. **Explanation:** Correct answer is A. *E. coli* is characterized as a gram-negative, lactose fermenting rod or bacilli. It is the most common pathogen (eg, 75–95%), associated with uncomplicated UTIs followed by other organisms in the Enterobacteriaceae family (eg, *Proteus mirabilis* and *Klebsiella pneumoniae*).[1] *A. baumanii* and *S. maltophilia* are characterized as nonlactose-fermenting gram-negative rods and uncommonly associated with uncomplicated UTIs. *S. aureus* is characterized as coagulase-positive, gram-positive cocci. The presence of *S. aureus* in the urine warrants further assessment since this is not a normal etiology for uncomplicated UTIs and could represent a hematogenously spread infection. Remember, UTIs are caused by the ascending spread of an organism into the genitourinary tract. *E. faecalis* is characterized as gamma hemolytic gram-positive cocci in pairs and chains.

6. **Explanation:** Correct answer is B. Although susceptible, the patient has an allergy to trimethoprim-sulfamethoxazole. Amoxicillin and cephalexin also demonstrate susceptibility; however, beta-lactams have lower rates of efficacy and require longer durations of therapy that may lead to more adverse effects.[1] In some scenarios it may be necessary to use amoxicillin or cephalexin, but VZ does not have any contraindications to nitrofurantoin. The goal is to use a narrow-spectrum agent to treat the *E. coli*–associated cystitis and amoxicillin, nitrofurantoin, and cephalexin are viable options. The spectrum of activity increases from amoxicillin to cephalexin and nitrofurantoin. Nitrofurantoin may demonstrate activity against multi-drug-resistant organisms (eg, ESBL-producing Enterobacteriaceae, MRSA, and VRE).[7]

7. **Explanation:** Correct answers are B, C, and E. Treatment of a urinary tract infection with phenazopyridine should not exceed 2 days because there is a lack of evidence that the combined administration of it with an antibacterial provides greater benefit than administration of the antibacterial alone after 2 days.[8] In addition, phenazopyridine is a urinary analgesic used to provide relief for dysuria and are more beneficial in patients with dysuria without a UTI.[2,8] The use of phenazopyridine beyond the recommended 2-day duration can increase the risk of side effects. Headache, rash, pruritus, gastrointestinal disturbance, and an anaphylactoid-like reaction have been reported.[8] Methemoglobinemia, hemolytic anemia, and renal and hepatic toxicity have also been reported, but this was associated with extended or chronic use. The use of phenazopyridine as an analgesic can hide or mask symptoms of the UTI that may indicate it is not improving.

REFERENCES

1. Gupta K, Hooton TM, Naber KG, et al. International clinical practice guidelines for the treatment of acute uncomplicated cystitis and pyelonephritis in women. *Clin Infect Dis*. 2011;52:e103-e120.

2. Sobel JD, Kaye D. Urinary tract infections. In Mandell GL, Bennett JE, Dolin R, eds. *Mandell, Douglas, and Bennett's Principles and Practice of Infectious Diseases*. Philadelphia, PA: Churchill Livingstone; 2010. Available at http://search.ebscohost.com/login.aspx?direct=true&db=nlebk&AN=458761&site=eds-live.

3. Simerville JA, Maxted WC, Pahira JJ. Urinalysis: a comprehensive review. *Am Fam Physician*. 2006;74:1153-1162.

4. Hooton TM, Winter C, Tiu F, et al. Randomized comparative trial and cost analysis of 3-day antimicrobial regimens for treatment of acute cystitis in women. *JAMA*. 1995;273:41-45.

5. Gupta K, Hooton TM, Roberts PL, et al. Short-course nitrofurantoin for the treatment of acute uncomplicated cystitis in women. *Arch Intern Med*. 2007;167:2207-2212.

6. Stein GE. Comparison of single-dose fosfomycin and a 7-day course of nitrofurantoin in female patients with uncomplicated urinary tract infection. *Clin Ther*. 1999; 21:1864-1872.

7. Huttner A, Stewardson A. Nitrofurans: Nitrofurazone, furazidine, and nitrofurantoin. In M. L. Grayson, ed. *Kucers' The Use of Antibiotics*. Boca Raton, FL: CRC Press; 2018. Available at https://online.vitalsource.com/#/books/9781351648158/cfi/6/260!/4/616/2@0:54.4

8. Pyridium (phenoazopyridine) [package insert]. Bridgewater, NJ: Gemini Laboratories, LLC; 2019.

8 Pyelonephritis

Marylee V. Worley

PATIENT PRESENTATION

Chief Complaint

"I have severe back pain and it hurts when I urinate."

History of Present Illness

KJ is a 58-year-old female who presents to the emergency department (ED) with complaints of fever, chills, dysuria, urgency, and back pain. Upon physical exam CVA tenderness is noted; no other significant physical findings. She has a fever of 101.2°F; however, she is hemodynamically stable in the ED.

Past Medical History

Hypertension × 10 years, congestive heart failure, hyperlipidemia, type 2 diabetes mellitus

Surgical History

None

Social History

Married, lives at home with husband and has 2 adult children who do not live at home

Allergies

Penicillins (reported a rash as a child)

Home Medications

Lisinopril 40 mg PO daily
Carvedilol 6.25 mg PO BID
Furosemide 20 mg PO daily
Atorvastatin 40 mg PO daily
Metformin 500 mg PO BID

Physical Examination

▶ *Vital Signs*

Temp 101.2°F, P 89, RR 18 breaths per minute, BP 139/73 mm Hg, Ht 5′4″, Wt 78 kg

▶ *General*

Mild distress, nontoxic appearing

▶ *HEENT*

Atraumatic, pupils equal round and reactive to light and accommodation, moist mucosa, normal pharynx, normal tonsils and adenoids, normal tongue

▶ *Pulmonary*

Normal chest wall expansion; no rales, no rhonchi, no wheezing

▶ *Cardiovascular*

Regular rate and rhythm, no murmurs, no gallops, normal S1 and S2

▶ *Abdomen*

Soft, non-tender, non-distended, normal bowel sounds in all quadrants, no hepatosplenomegaly

▶ *Genitourinary*

No incontinence, complains of dysuria

▶ *Neurology*

No headache, focal numbness or weakness, dizziness, or seizures

▶ *Musculoskeletal*

CVA tenderness noted, normal ROM in upper and lower extremities, no swelling, no joint erythema; Integumentary: warm, dry, pink, with no rash, purpura, or petechia

Laboratory Findings

Na = 140 mEq/L	BUN = 26 mg/dL	Hgb = 13.2 g/dL
K = 3.8 mEq/L	SCr = 1.0 mg/dL	Hct = 36%
Cl = 98 mEq/L	Glucose = 161 mg/dL	Plt = $280 \times 10^3/mm^3$
CO_2 = 26 mEq/L		WBC = $14.2 \times 10^3/mm^3$

QUESTIONS

1. What laboratory tests are recommended for patients with suspected pyelonephritis?
   A. Urine culture
   B. CRP
   C. ESR
   D. Urine osmolality

2. What is a likely sign or symptom of pyelonephritis?
   A. Back pain
   B. Dysuria
   C. Fever
   D. All of the above

3. Which of the following findings in KJ's urinalysis are consistent with urinary tract infections?
   A. Many epithelial cells
   B. Negative nitrite
   C. Large leukocyte esterase
   D. Yellow color

Urinalysis from KJ

Component	Value	Range & Units
Color	Yellow	
Transparency	Cloudy	
Specific gravity	1.009	1.005–1.030
pH	5.0	5.0–8.0
Protein	Negative	Negative, mg/dL
Glucose	Negative	Negative, mg/dL
Ketones	Negative	Negative, mg/dL
Bilirubin	Negative	Negative
Blood	Negative	Negative
Nitrite	Negative	Negative
Urobilinogen	0.2	0.2–1.0 mg/dL
Leukocyte esterase	Large	Negative
WBC	>50	None seen/HPF
RBC	0–2	None seen/HPF
Bacteria	Many	None seen/HPF
Epithelial cells	Many	None seen/HPF

Hospital Antibiogram

4. Which empiric antimicrobial therapy is most appropriate for KJ based on the most likely pathogen and the hospital antibiogram provided above?
   A. Fosfomycin 3 g oral once
   B. Nitrofurantoin 100 mg orally twice daily for 5 days
   C. Levofloxacin 500 mg IV every 24 hours
   D. Ceftriaxone 1 g IV every 24 hours

Gram-Negative Isolates (Data expressed in % susceptibility)	# of Isolates	Ampicillin/ Sulbactam	Aztreonam	Cefazolin	Cefepime	Ceftazidime	Ceftriaxone	Ertapenem	Gentamicin	Levofloxacin	Meropenem	Nitrofurantoin	Piperacillin/ Tazobactam	Tigecycline	Tobramycin	Trimethoprim/ Sulfamethoxazole
Acinetobacter baumannii	80	87	/	/	62	61	/	/	71	69	74	/	73	81	86	64
Citrobacter freundii	45	/	86	/	100	82	86	100	91	89	100	91	88	89	91	75
Citrobacter koseri	69	/	100	97	100	100	100	100	100	100	100	97	97	100	98	97
Enterobacter aerogenes	63	/	82	/	100	82	85	100	95	98	100	/	86	95	94	97
Enterobacter cloacae complex	149	/	87	/	95	87	85	97	93	88	97	58	87	94	92	85
Escherichia coli	3534	45	81	76	82	81	81	100	81	48	100	94	93	100	78	
Klebsiella oxytoca	98	76	99	71	99	99	99	100	99	97	100	96	94	100	99	53
Klebsiella pneumoniae	661	66	80	75	79	79	79	98	87	77	98	38	82	90	80	97
Morganella morganii	127	/	96	/	95	93	91	100	80	56	100	/	98	/	79	76
Proteus mirabilis	608	80	91	80	92	92	92	100	93	68	99	/	99	/	94	42
Providencia stuartii	52	/	100	/	100	98	100	98	/	33	100	/	98	/	/	61
Pseudomonas aeruginosa	637	/	/	/	84	85	/	/	87	70	88	/	89	/	95	52
Serratia marcescens	85	/	89	/	92	89	91	92	95	88	92	/	/	88	80	98

The forward slash "/" indicates "no clinically relevant activity of that antibiotic against that organism."

5. If preliminary blood cultures report lactose-fermenting, gram-negative bacilli, what is the most common organism associated with UTIs which is known to have these characteristics?
   A. *Escherichia coli*
   B. *Pseudomonas aeruginosa*
   C. *Stenotrophomonas maltophilia*
   D. *Haemophilus influenzae*

6. If the culture returns with the below susceptibility results, which antimicrobial is the most appropriate option for KJ?
   A. Tigecycline
   B. Ertapenem
   C. Fosfomycin
   D. Piperacillin/Tazobactam

Microbiology Results: Blood cultures (2/2 collected on day 1): *Escherichia coli*

	MIC (mcg/mL)	Interpretation
Levofloxacin	0.25	S
Cefazolin	>64	R
Ceftriaxone	>64	R
Cefepime	>64	R
ESBL	+	Positive
Piperacillin/Tazobactam	8	S
Tigecycline	0.5	S
Meropenem	0.5	S
Gentamicin	1	S

Urine Cultures: *Escherichia coli* (same as above)

7. Based on the same culture results above, which of the following antimicrobial options would be appropriate if the patient was allergic to carbapenems?
   A. Moxifloxacin
   B. Levofloxacin
   C. Meropenem
   D. Ceftriaxone

8. What is the appropriate duration of treatment for uncomplicated pyelonephritis?
   A. 7–10 days
   B. 14 days
   C. 3 days
   D. Both A or B could be appropriate depending on the antimicrobial prescribed

ANSWERS

1. **Explanation:** The correct answer is A. Urine samples that are a clean-catch, mid-stream or from a catheterized urine sample should be sent for culture and susceptibility testing. This should be performed for all patients with pyelonephritis in order to tailor the empiric therapy based on the resistance pattern of the patient-specific uropathogen. CRP (C-reactive protein) and ESR (erythrocyte sedimentation rate) are both non-specific markers of inflammation that can be detected in the blood; however, both are not utilized for the management of patients with pyelonephritis. The response to therapy should be assessed and measured based on resolution of the patient's signs and symptoms of the infection based on their original clinical presentation (eg, If the patient presented febrile initially, has the patient defervesced?). Urine osmolality is not utilized for the management of urinary tract infections and normally part of the diagnostic workup for certain electrolyte disturbances such as hyponatremia in a euvolemic patient.

2. **Explanation:** The correct answer is D. Back pain, dysuria, and fever are all potential signs or symptoms of pyelonephritis. Upper urinary tract infections involve the kidney and are referred to as pyelonephritis, which can lead to patients experiencing lower flank pain that is often expressed by patients more generally as back pain. The physical exam finding of costovertebral angle (CVA) tenderness may be documented, which represents pain around the kidneys. Symptoms from cystitis are often also present in patients presenting with pyelonephritis as most infections are ascending, meaning they travel from the bladder to the kidneys. Lower tract infections including cystitis (bladder), urethritis (urethra), prostatitis (prostate gland), and epididymitis will lead to symptoms such as dysuria, urgency, frequency, nocturia, and suprapubic heaviness. In elderly patients presenting with UTIs, there may not be specific urinary symptoms, but they may present with altered mental status, change in eating habits, or gastrointestinal symptoms.

3. **Explanation:** The correct answer is C. The finding of large leukocyte esterase is consistent with urinary tract infections as it is an indicator that the white blood cells are actively making enzymes in response to a possible infection. Leukocyte esterase is found in primary neutrophil granules and indicates the presence of WBCs, which when detected in urine is called pyuria. The detection of WBCs upon microscopic examination is also indicative of pyuria. The nitrite test is used to detect the presence of nitrate-reducing bacteria in the urine (eg, *E. coli*). Nitrites can be negative even if there is an infection; however, a positive nitrite would be more consistent with a UTI due to the fact that the most common organisms that cause UTI (Enterobacteriaceae) are normally nitrite reducers. The finding of many epithelial cells is indicative that this was not a "clean catch," which is neither consistent nor nonconsistent with a UTI as it normally represents a contaminated sample. Obtaining a midstream clean catch is the preferred method for urine collection for urine cultures. Patients need to be instructed on the proper collection technique, which involves cleaning (normally with a moist wipe) the urethral opening area and discarding the initial 20 to 30 mL of urine, followed by collection of the urine specimen. The color of the urine is not normally considered with the diagnosis of a UTI.

4. **Explanation:** The correct answer is D. Ceftriaxone is the most appropriate empiric therapy for treatment of pyelonephritis based on the susceptibility rates.[1] The most common organism that causes uncomplicated UTIs is *Escherichia coli,* and according to this antibiogram, *Escherichia coli* is only 48% susceptible to levofloxacin and this is why it would not be the correct answer. Nitrofurantoin and fosfomycin orally are both only indicated for treatment of cystitis due to the lack of sufficient concentrations in the kidneys that would be necessary to treat pyelonephritis.

5. **Explanation:** The correct answer is A. *Escherichia coli* is the most common organism to cause an uncomplicated UTI. All four answer choices listed share the morphology of gram-negative bacilli. *Haemophilus influenzae* is more commonly associated with upper respiratory tract infections and not a normal pathogen for UTIs. *Stenotrophomonas maltophilia* is associated with infections related to devices or indwelling catheters due to biofilm formation. *Stenotrophomonas maltophilia* is not commonly implicated in an uncomplicated UTI and can be rarely involved in nosocomial UTIs. *Pseudomonas aeruginosa* can cause UTIs; however, it is not one of the most common causes of uncomplicated UTIs, whereas empiric coverage for *Pseudomonas aeruginosa* could be considered in patients with obstruction, foreign body, chronic indwelling catheter, or complicated UTIs.

6. **Explanation:** The correct answer is B. Ertapenem is the correct answer based on the culture findings of ESBL-producing *E. coli.* This patient's allergy to penicillin, although it was not reported as anaphylactic, would make piperacillin/tazobactam not an acceptable choice, in addition to growing evidence that demonstrates inferiority compared to carbapenems for treatment of bloodstream infections caused by ESBL-producing organisms.[2] Tigecycline, although reporting as susceptible, is not appropriate to treat infections in the urinary tract due to the pharmacokinetic concerns with using tigecycline for UTI as only 22% of the total dose is excreted unchanged. Fosfomycin is currently only available orally in the United States, and the oral formulation does not achieve high enough concentrations in the blood to treat bacteremia.

7. **Explanation:** The correct answer is B. Levofloxacin would be appropriate for invasive ESBL infections that show susceptibility, in the absence of the option to treat with the drug of choice for this type of infection, which is a carbapenem. Meropenem is a carbapenem, so this would not be appropriate in patients with a carbapenem allergy. Ceftriaxone is not listed as a susceptible option according to this patient's culture results and moxifloxacin is not appropriate for treatment of UTIs due to low urinary concentrations.

8. **Explanation:** The correct answer is D. Depending on the antimicrobial prescribed, there is evidence to support a treatment duration with fluoroquinolones for 7 days of treatment and trimethoprim–sulfamethoxazole for 14 days or a beta-lactam for 10 to 14 days of treatment.[1]

REFERENCES

1. Gupta K, Hooton TM, Naber KG, et al. International clinical practice guidelines for the treatment of acute uncomplicated cystitis and pyelonephritis in women: a 2010 update by the IDSA and ESMID. *Clin Infect Dis.* 2011;52(5):e103-e120.
2. Harris PNA, Tambyah PA, Lye DC, et al. Effect of piperacillin-tazobactam vs meropenem on 30-day mortality for patients with *E. coli* or *Klebsiella pneumoniae* bloodstream infection and ceftriaxone resistance: A randomized clinical trial. *JAMA.* 2018;320(10):984-994.

9 Bacterial Meningitis

Jonathan C. Cho

PATIENT PRESENTATION

Chief Complaint

"I have severe headaches and fevers."

History of Present Illness

DJ is a 54-year-old Caucasian female who presents to the emergency department with worsening headache, neck pain, and back pain of 2 days duration. She also complains of low-grade fevers and chills that developed over the past 24 hours. Her son, who is present during her exam, states that she seems more lethargic and has difficulty maintaining her balance. In addition, she reports 3 to 4 episodes of nausea and vomiting.

Past Medical History

CHF, COPD, HTN, epilepsy, stroke, hypothyroidism, anxiety

Surgical History

Hysterectomy, cholecystectomy

Family History

Father had HTN and passed away from a stroke 4 years ago; mother has type II DM and epilepsy; brother has HTN

Social History

Divorced but lives with her two sons who are currently attending college. Smokes ½ ppd × 27 years and drinks alcohol occasionally.

Allergies

NKDA

Home Medications

Advair 250 mcg/50 mcg 1 puff BID
Albuterol metered-dose-inhaler 2 puffs q4h PRN shortness of breath
Alprazolam 0.5 mg PO daily
Aspirin 81 mg PO daily
Atorvastatin 20 mg PO daily
Carvedilol 6.25 mg PO BID
Citalopram 20 mg PO daily
Divalproex sodium 500 mg PO BID
Furosemide 20 mg PO daily
Levothyroxine 88 mcg PO daily
Levetiracetam 500 mg PO BID
Lisinopril 20 mg PO daily

Physical Examination

▶ Vital Signs

Temp 101.2°F, P 72, RR 23 breaths per minute, BP 162/87 mm Hg, pO$_2$ 91%, Ht 5'3", Wt 56.4 kg

▶ General

Lethargic, female with dizziness and in mild to moderate distress.

▶ HEENT

Normocephalic, atraumatic, PERRLA, EOMI, pale or dry mucous membranes and conjunctiva, poor dentition

▶ Pulmonary

Diminished breath sounds and crackles bilaterally.

▶ Cardiovascular

NSR, no m/r/g

▶ Abdomen

Soft, non-distended, non-tender, bowel sounds hyperactive

▶ Genitourinary

Normal female genitalia, no complaints of dysuria or hematuria

▶ Neurology

Lethargic, oriented to place and person, (–) Brudzinski's sign, (+) Kernig's sign

▶ Extremities

Pedal edema on lower extremities, petechial lesions on lower and upper extremities

▶ *Back*

Tenderness to palpation on lower lumbar region

Laboratory Findings

Na = 136 mEq/L   Hgb = 14.5 g/dL   Ca = 8.1 mg/dL

K = 4.1 mEq/L   Hct = 38%   Mg = 2.2 mg/dL

Cl = 98 mEq/L   Plt = 132×10^3/mm³   Phos = 4.6 mg/dL

CO_2 = 26 mEq/L   WBC = 8×10^3/mm³   AST = 24 IU/L

BUN = 26 mg/dL   Trop < 0.01 ng/mL   ALT = 22 IU/L

SCr = 1.66 mg/dL   CK = 3 ng/mL   T Bili = 1.8 mg/dL

Glu = 168 mg/dL   BNP = 64 pg/mL   Alk Phos = 76 IU/L

▶ *CT Head*

Diffuse hypodensity in the left lentiform nucleus, possibly from a previous stroke

▶ *Blood Cultures*

Pending

▶ *LP/CSF Analysis*

Pending

▶ *CSF Gram Stain*

Pending

QUESTIONS

1. Which laboratory test(s) help identify a patient with bacterial meningitis?
   A. Positive Gram stain of CSF
   B. Low CSF glucose (<40 mg/dL)
   C. High percentage of neutrophils in CSF
   D. All of the above

2. DJ's CSF analysis revealed WBC 1750 cells/mm³ with 88% neutrophils, 330 mg/dL protein, and glucose 40 mg/dL (plasma glucose 165 mg/dL). What is the most likely diagnosis for DJ?
   A. Community-acquired bacterial meningitis
   B. Healthcare-associated bacterial meningitis
   C. Viral meningitis
   D. Fungal meningitis

3. What is a likely sign or symptom of bacterial meningitis in DJ?
   A. Diminished breath sounds and crackles
   B. Pedal edema on lower extremities
   C. Severe headaches
   D. Dyspnea

4. Which empiric antimicrobial therapy is most appropriate for DJ?
   A. Ampicillin + cefotaxime
   B. Vancomycin + ampicillin + ceftriaxone
   C. Vancomycin + cefotaxime
   D. Vancomycin + cefepime

5. If the preliminary CSF Gram stain resulted in gram (+) bacilli, coverage against what pathogen should be included?
   A. *Streptococcus pneumoniae*
   B. *Listeria monocytogenes*
   C. *Haemophilus influenzae*
   D. *Neisseria meningitidis*

6. Once *Listeria monocytogenes* is isolated, what antimicrobial agent would you recommend for treatment of bacterial meningitis in DJ?
   A. Ampicillin 2 g IV q4h
   B. Ceftriaxone 1g IV q24h
   C. Meropenem 1g IV q8h
   D. Cefepime 1g IV q12h

7. What is the appropriate duration of treatment for bacterial meningitis caused by *Haemophilus influenzae*?
   A. 7 days
   B. 10–14 days
   C. 14–21 days
   D. ≥21 days

8. Which is true regarding dexamethasone use in bacterial meningitis?
   A. Should be administered empirically in patients with suspected pneumococcal meningitis
   B. Reduces inflammatory responses in the subarachnoid space, decreasing risk of neurologic sequelae due to bacterial meningitis
   C. May reduce antimicrobial penetration into CSF
   D. All of the above

ANSWERS

1. **Explanation:** The correct answer is D. A Gram stain examination of CSF allows for rapid identification of the causative bacterium with high rates of specificity. CSF analysis can also aid in the diagnosis of bacterial meningitis. Usual CSF findings in the setting of bacterial meningitis include low glucose (<40 mg/dL), elevated white blood cell count (>1000 cells/mm³), high percentage of neutrophils (>80%), and elevated protein (>200 mg/dL). In addition to these findings, elevated CSF lactate concentrations can help to distinguish between bacterial and viral (aseptic) meningitis. Blood cultures can also guide antimicrobial therapy, especially in patients whom lumbar puncture cannot be performed.

Meningitis CSF Laboratory Findings

	Normal	Bacterial	Viral	Fungal
WBC (cells/mm³)	<5	1000–5000	5–500	100–400
WBC differential	Monocytes	Neutrophils (>80%)	Lymphocytes (>50%)	Lymphocytes (>50%)
Protein (mg/dL)	<50	Elevated (100–500)	Slightly elevated	Elevated (60–150)
Glucose (mg/dL)	45–80	Decreased (<45)	Normal	Decreased (<45)
CSF/blood glucose ratio	0.5–0.6	Decreased (<0.4)	Normal	Decreased (<0.4)

2. **Explanation:** The correct answer is A. DJ's CSF analysis is consistent with bacterial meningitis with elevated WBC (neutrophil predominant), elevated protein, decreased glucose, and decreased CSF/blood glucose ratio (rules out answers C and D). Health care–associated bacterial meningitis is associated with head trauma, neurosurgical procedures, or placement of ventricular catheters (rules out answer B).

3. **Explanation:** The correct answer is C. Fever, nuchal rigidity, headache, and altered mental status are common symptoms associated with bacterial meningitis. Other classic symptoms include Brudzinski's sign (flexion of the hips when knees are flexed), Kernig's sign (inability to extend knee when hips are flexed), and purpuric and/or petechial skin lesions. Presentation can vary with risk factors and age, including clinical manifestations such as bulging fontanelle (in infants) and neurologic complications (such as ataxia or convulsions). DJ presents with symptoms consistent with bacterial meningitis: headaches, fever, neck and back pain, lethargy, and (+) Kernig's sign. DJ's diminished breath sounds and crackles are likely due to her COPD, pedal edema due to her CHF, and dyspnea due to her CHF or COPD (rules out answers A, B, and D).

4. **Explanation:** The correct answer is B. In patients more than 50 years of age, the recommended antimicrobial therapy is vancomycin, ampicillin, and a third-generation cephalosporin (ceftriaxone or cefotaxime), as the most common bacterial pathogens are *Streptococcus pneumoniae*, *Neisseria meningitidis*, aerobic gram (–) bacilli, and *Listeria monocytogenes*. Ceftriaxone is active against *S. pneumoniae* and gram (–) organisms, ampicillin is added for *L. monocytogenes* coverage, and vancomycin is used to provide additional *S. pneumoniae* coverage until susceptibilities are known. Answer A is appropriate empiric treatment for patients less than 1 month of age (ampicillin, in combination with either cefotaxime or an aminoglycoside, is recommended, as *L. monocytogenes* is a potential pathogen in this age group). Ceftriaxone should not be used in patients younger than 1 month as it can cause biliary sludging and hyperbilirubinemia. Answer C is appropriate in patients 1 month of age to 50 years of age as *L. monocytogenes* is not considered a common pathogen in this age group. Answer D is appropriate in patients with health care–associated bacterial meningitis as resistant gram-negative bacilli (i.e. *Pseudomonas aeruginosa*) is a potential pathogen requiring the use of cefepime.[1]

5. **Explanation:** The correct answer is B. Due to the increased rates of pathogenicity, a CSF Gram stain showing gram (+) diplococci often suggests *Streptococcus pneumoniae*, gram (–) diplococci suggests *Neisseria meningitidis*, gram (–) coccobacilli suggests *Haemophilus influenzae*, and gram (+) bacilli suggests *Listeria monocytogenes*. *L. monocytogenes* can cause bacterial meningitis primarily in the elderly, newborns, and immunocompromised patients.

6. **Explanation:** The correct answer is A. Current guidelines recommend four antimicrobial options against isolated *L. monocytogenes* in cases of bacterial meningitis: ampicillin or penicillin G as standards of treatment while trimethoprim-sulfamethoxazole or meropenem serve as alternative regimens.[1] Ampicillin has excellent activity against *L. monocytogenes* and remains the preferred antimicrobial option. Cephalosporins are not active against *Listeria* sp. ruling out answers B and D. Meropenem is an option, but due to the drug–drug interaction with divalproex sodium (meropenem lowers divalproex concentrations below therapeutic ranges; therefore, increasing the risk of breakthrough seizures), it is not preferred. Additionally, higher doses of intravenous antimicrobials are needed for the treatment of bacterial meningitis (ruling out answers B, C, and D).

7. **Explanation:** The correct answer is A. Current guidelines recommend 7 days of treatment for *Neisseria meningitidis* and *Haemophilus influenzae*, 10 to 14 days for *Streptococcus pneumoniae*, 14 to 21 days for *Streptococcus agalactiae*, 21 days for aerobic gram-negative bacilli, and ≥21 days for *Listeria monocytogenes* when isolated in the setting of bacterial meningitis.[1] Although these recommendations are available, treatment duration should depend on individual patient response.

8. **Explanation:** The correct answer is D. Dexamethasone therapy is recommended as adjunctive therapy to antimicrobial

therapy in patients with suspected or proven pneumococcal meningitis. Dexamethasone should be administered 10 to 20 minutes before the first dose of antimicrobial therapy and only continued in patients with bacterial meningitis due to *Streptococcus pneumoniae*. In patients who have already received antimicrobial therapy, use of dexamethasone is not recommended, as it is not likely to improve patient outcomes. Adjunctive dexamethasone therapy may decrease inflammatory responses in the subarachnoid space and reduce neurologic sequelae from bacterial meningitis. Although the benefits are known, clinical controversy regarding adjunctive dexamethasone use exists as dexamethasone may reduce inflammatory responses that aid in CSF penetration of certain antimicrobials, such as vancomycin.

REFERENCE

1. Tunkel AR, Hartman BJ, Kaplan SL, et al. Practice guidelines for the management of bacterial meningitis. *Clin Infect Dis*. 2004;39:1267-1284.

10 Viral Encephalitis

Ann Lloyd

PATIENT PRESENTATION

Chief Complaint

Altered mental status and fever

History of Present Illness

GA is a 23-year-old Caucasian female who presents to the emergency department with her parents who report that she has been behaving abnormally over the past several days. They report that she was withdrawn and would not speak. She has complained of a sore throat.

Past Medical History

Depression

Surgical History

None

Family History

Mother with HTN and depression, father with type II DM

Social History

Smokes ½ ppd × 5 years and drinks alcohol socially

Allergies

NKDA

Home Medications

Fluoxetine 40 mg PO once daily

Physical Examination

▶ Vital Signs

Temp 100.4°F, P 141, RR 31 breaths per minute, BP 151/89 mm Hg, pO_2 98%, Ht 5′6″, Wt 60 kg

▶ General

Febrile, following limited commands, but in no acute distress

▶ HEENT

+3 tonsils without exudate, normocephalic, atraumatic, EOMI, PERRLA

▶ Pulmonary

Clear to auscultation bilaterally

▶ Cardiovascular

Tachycardic, regular rhythm, no m/r/g

▶ Abdomen

Soft, non-distended, no masses

▶ Neurology

Oriented to person and situation, follows some instructions and nods head but does not speak

▶ Extremities

Warm and dry, no edema, no rashes, ulcers, or lesions

Laboratory Findings

Na = 129 mEq/L	Hgb = 12.4 g/dL	Ca = 8.6 mg/dL
K = 3.5 mEq/L	Hct = 38%	AST = 26 IU/L
Cl = 97 mEg/L	Plt = 248 × 10^3/mm³	ALT = 15 IU/L
CO_2 = 21 mEq/L	WBC = 13.5 × 10^3/mm³	T Bili = 0.6 mg/dL
BUN = 13 mg/dL		Alk Phos = 51 IU/L
SCr = 0.88 mg/dL		
Glu = 112 mg/dL		

▶ CSF Analysis

Colorless, hazy; RBC 0 cells/mm³, WBC 426 cells/mm³, 10% segs, 72% lymphs, 18% monos

▶ CSF Protein

75 mg/dL

▶ CSF Glucose

61 mg/dL

▶ CSF Gram Stain/Culture

Pending

▶ Throat Culture

Pending

> ## CSF Meningitis Panel by PCR (see table for contents of the panel)

Pending

CSF Meningitis Panel by PCR		
Bacteria	**Viruses**	**Yeast**
Escherichia coli	Cytomegalovirus	*Cryptococcus neoformans/ gatti*
Haemophilus influenzae	Enterovirus	
Listeria monocytogenes	Herpes simplex virus 1	
Neisseria meningitidis	Herpes simplex virus 2	
Streptococcus agalactiae	Human herpesvirus 6	
Streptococcus pneumoniae	Human parechovirus	
	Varicella zoster virus	

> ## CXR

Normal

> ## MRI Brain

Abnormal restricted diffusion, cortical edema, and vasogenic edema involving the anterior temporal lobe, hippocampus, insular ribbon, and medial thalamus

QUESTIONS

1. Which laboratory findings in this patient make the diagnosis of viral encephalitis most likely?
   A. Lymphocyte predominance on the CSF differential
   B. Slightly elevated CSF protein
   C. Normal CSF glucose
   D. All of the above

2. Which empiric therapy is most appropriate for GA while awaiting the CSF Gram stain and culture?
   A. Acyclovir
   B. Acyclovir, ceftriaxone, and vancomycin
   C. Ampicillin, ceftriaxone, and vancomycin
   D. Acyclovir, ampicillin, ceftriaxone, and vancomycin

3. Which of the following acyclovir regimens should be started for GA?
   A. Acyclovir 400 mg PO five times daily
   B. Acyclovir 800 mg PO five times daily
   C. Acyclovir 600 mg IV every 8 hours
   D. Acyclovir 900 mg IV every 8 hours

4. GA's meningitis PCR results return with no positive findings. What is the most appropriate change to her anti-infective regimen?
   A. Continue acyclovir, ceftriaxone, and vancomycin
   B. Continue acyclovir, but discontinue vancomycin and ceftriaxone
   C. Discontinue acyclovir, but continue ceftriaxone and vancomycin
   D. Discontinue acyclovir, ceftriaxone, and vancomycin

5. Three days later, GA's HSV PCR returns with a positive result confirming the diagnosis of HSV encephalitis. Her CSF Gram stain is negative and there is no growth on the CSF culture. What changes should be made to her anti-infective regimen now?
   A. Continue acyclovir, ceftriaxone, and vancomycin
   B. Continue acyclovir, but discontinue vancomycin and ceftriaxone
   C. Discontinue acyclovir, but continue ceftriaxone and vancomycin
   D. Discontinue acyclovir, ceftriaxone, and vancomycin

6. What is the appropriate duration of treatment for viral encephalitis caused by HSV?
   A. 5 days
   B. 7 days
   C. 10 days
   D. 14–21 days

7. Which of the following adverse effects may be seen while GA is receiving intravenous acyclovir?
   A. Myopathy
   B. Nephrotoxicity
   C. Ototoxicty
   D. Thrombocytopenia

ANSWERS

1. **Explanation:** The correct answer is D. It is often difficult to distinguish viral encephalitis from bacterial meningitis especially while awaiting the CSF Gram stain and culture. However, in this case, the lymphocyte predominance on the CSF differential along with the slightly elevated CSF protein but normal CSF glucose all point more toward a viral cause of this patient's meningitis. In the table below, the differences between bacterial and viral CSF findings are compared to normal CSF.

Mean Values of Components of Normal and Abnormal CSF

Variable	Normal	Bacterial	Viral
Opening pressure	60–220 mm H_2O	Increased (>250 mm H_2O)	Rarely increased
WBC (cells/mm³)	UP to 5	1,000–5,000	100–500
Dominant cell type	Lymphocytes	Neutrophils	Lymphocytes
Protein (mg/dL)	20–60 mg/dL	Usually increased (100–500 mg/dL)	Normal/slightly increased
Glucose (mg/dL)	Two-thirds of serum	Low (<40 mg/dL or 40% of concurrent serum)	Normal

2. **Explanation:** The correct answer is B. While awaiting the CSF Gram stain and culture results, empiric therapy should be started as soon as possible providing coverage against both bacterial and viral meningitis. Because this patient is between the ages of 1 month and 50 years old, she is at risk for the following most common types of bacterial meningitis: *Streptococcus pneumoniae, Neisseria meningitidis,* and *Haemophilus influenza.*[1] Additionally, based on her presentation and laboratory findings, there is a suspicion for viral causes of her infection. The most common viral pathogens include herpes simplex virus (HSV), West Nile virus, enteroviruses, and other herpesviruses. In order to provide coverage against all possible organisms, the patient should be immediately started on acyclovir, ceftriaxone, and vancomycin (rules out answer A) pending the results of the CSF Gram stain and culture as well as the CSF meningitis panel. Ampicillin should be added to empiric therapy regimens for patients younger than 1 month, older than age 50, or immunocompromised patients to provide coverage against *Listeria monocytogenes* (rules out answers C and D).

3. **Explanation:** The correct answer is C. For patients receiving acyclovir for suspected HSV encephalitis, intravenous acyclovir is the drug of choice (rules out answers A and B). For adult patients, the usual dose is 10 mg/kg IV every 8 hours (rules out answer D). In neonates, the dose is increased to 20 mg/kg IV every 8 hours to improve outcomes and prevent relapses. These same benefits are not seen when the dose is increased in adult patients. There is some controversy surrounding the weight that should be used to dose acyclovir in obese patients. Historically, the ideal body weight was used to dose acyclovir. However, there is concern that this may result in underdosing of obese patients. Some clinicians may elect to use adjusted body weight for dosing in obese patients.[2]

4. **Explanation:** The correct answer is A. Despite the meningitis PCR returning with no positive findings, there is still a very high suspicion for a central nervous system infection.[1] Therefore, all empiric therapy should be continued pending further laboratory studies. In this patient's case, the MRI findings which include edema in the temporal lobe are strongly suggestive of HSV encephalitis. Further, altered mental status is more common in encephalitis compared to meningitis. Finally, the initial HSV PCR (which is included in the meningitis PCR) may be negative and should be repeated. Until these results can be repeated, all empiric therapy should be continued pending the CSF Gram stain and culture and the repeat HSV PCR.

5. **Explanation:** The correct answer is B. Now that the HSV PCR is positive and there is no bacterial growth on the CSF culture, the vancomycin and ceftriaxone can be discontinued. Intravenous acyclovir alone should be continued to treat the HSV infection.

6. **Explanation:** The correct answer is D. According to current guidelines, intravenous acyclovir should be continued for 14 to 21 days.[1] The actual duration of treatment should be determined once individual patient characteristics are taken into consideration and could be longer than 21 days in certain situations.

7. **Explanation:** The correct answer is B. Although oral formulations of acyclovir are usually well tolerated, the intravenous form requires specific monitoring. In addition to neurotoxicity, practitioners should monitor patients for changes in renal function (rules out answers A, C, and D). Serum creatinine levels may increase while on therapy. With high doses or in patients with renal insufficiency, acyclovir may crystallize in the renal tubules. Dose adjustments should occur for patients with renal dysfunction, and prehydration with intravenous fluids may decrease the risk of nephrotoxicity.

REFERENCES

1. Tunkel AR, Glaser CA, Bloch KC, et al. The management of encephalitis: clinical practice guidelines by the Infectious Diseases Society of America. *Clin Infect Dis.* 2008;47:303-327.
2. Wong A, Pickering AJ, Potoski BA. Dosing practices of intravenous acyclovir for herpes encephalitis in obesity: results of a pharmacist survey. *J Pharm Pract.* 2017;30(3):324-328.

11 Infective Endocarditis

Rachel A. Foster   P. Brandon Bookstaver

PATIENT PRESENTATION

Chief Complaint

Headache, fevers, and chills

History of Present Illness

GR is a 68-year-old woman with a notable past medical history of rheumatoid arthritis on infliximab and a prosthetic aortic valve, who was brought to the emergency department (ED) after her family found her extremely lethargic and confused at home. She had been complaining of fevers, chills, headache, and neck pain for 2 days prior to presentation, and as per the patient's family had steadily become less and less communicative. Otherwise the patient has had no major medical issues in the last year since her aortic valve replacement.

Past Medical History

CAD, depression, type II DM, eczema, HTN, fibromyalgia, severe aortic stenosis with valve replacement

Surgical History

Bioprosthetic aortic valve replacement (10 months ago), S2–S4 diskectomy (4 years ago), tubal ligation (>15 years ago), cholecystectomy (>15 years ago)

Family History

Father passed away from HF; mother has type II DM, HTN, and h/o stroke; sister has type II DM, COPD, and HTN

Social History

Widowed, lives by herself, never used alcohol, former smoker (quit 10 years ago)

Allergies

Hydrocodone/acetaminophen (vomiting)

Home Medications

Aspirin DR tablet 81 mg PO daily
Atorvastatin 20 mg PO daily
Fluoxetine 40 mg PO daily
Glimepiride 4 mg PO daily
Infliximab 3 mg/kg IV every 2 months
Lisinopril 10 mg PO daily
Pregabalin 75 mg PO BID
Triamcinolone 0.1% lotion topical BID
Vitamin D3 5,000 IU PO daily

Physical Examination

▶ Vital Signs

Temp 102.1°F (tympanic), HR 112 bpm, RR 19 breaths per minute, BP 91/52 mm Hg, SpO$_2$ 97% (on room air), Ht 165 cm, Wt 91 kg, BMI 33.4 kg/m^2

▶ General

Lethargic, acutely ill appearing, appears stated age

▶ HEENT

Normocephalic, atraumatic, PERRLA, EOMI, faint conjunctival hemorrhage, non-icteric sclera, poor dentition, no erythema or swelling in the oropharynx

▶ Neck

No nuchal rigidity, tenderness to palpation on lower lumbar region

▶ Pulmonary

Clear to auscultation bilaterally, no wheezes or crackles

▶ Cardiovascular

Regular rate and rhythm, faint systolic murmur over the right base

▶ Abdomen

Soft, non-distended, no masses, no focal rebound or guarding, tenderness in the epigastric region to palpation

▶ Genitourinary

No complaints of dysuria or hematuria

▶ Neurology

AO × 1, no focal deficits, strength and sensation full and symmetric

► **Extremities**

Intact distal pulses, no LE edema

► **Skin**

Warm and diaphoretic

► **Back**

Tenderness to palpation on lower lumbar region

Laboratory Findings

Na = 124 mmol/L   BUN = 28 mg/dL   T bili: 1.9 mg/dL

K = 3.4 mmol/L   SCr = 1.4 mg/dL   Alk Phos = 96 unit/L

Cl = 88 mmol/L   Ca = 9.8 mg/dL   AST = 109 unit/L

CO_2 = 19 mmol/L   Protein, total = 7.9 g/dL   ALT = 92 unit/L

Glucose = 286 mg/dL   Albumin = 3.8 g/dL

Estimated CrCl: 36.47 mL/min; estimated GFR: 40 mL/min/1.73 m^2

WBC = 21.3 K/µL   Segs = 72%   Bands = 22%

Lymphocytes = 2%   Monocytes = 4%   Neutrophil, abs = 18.1 K/µL

Lymphocyte, abs = 0.4 K/µL   Monocyte, abs = 0.8 K/µL   MCHC = 33.8 g/dL

RBC = 3.74 × 10^6/µL   RDW SD = 42.4 fL   Hemoglobin = 11.5 g/dL

RDW = 13.5%   Hematocrit = 32.4%   Platelets = 86 K/µL

MCV = 86.5 fL   MPV = 10.8 fL   MCH = 29.3 pg

Lactic acid, venous: 2.5 mmol/L

Imaging

► **CT Head**

Unremarkable, no evidence of infarct or hemorrhagic stroke

► **CXR**

Indistinct central pulmonary vasculature, suggestive of pulmonary venous congestion but no radiographic evidence of pneumonia

► **Transthoracic Echocardiogram (TTE)**

LVEF 73% (±3%), normal RV systolic function, AV appears to be well seated with normal functioning and trace regurgitation, no pulmonary hypertension or pericardial effusion seen; the study is of adequate quality

ED Course

Blood cultures are drawn and GR undergoes a lumbar puncture. She is started on vancomycin, ceftriaxone, ampicillin, acyclovir, and dexamethasone for empiric treatment of meningitis/encephalitis while further workup is done in the setting of immunosuppression. The HSV PCR on the CSF returns negative and the acyclovir is discontinued. Shortly thereafter, her blood cultures (2/2 sets) flag positive and the Gram stain shows gram-positive cocci (GPC) in clusters. An hour later, rapid diagnostic technology confirms the GPCs in the blood cultures are methicillin-sensitive *Staphylococcus aureus* (MSSA). The CSF analysis also returns and reveals a CSF clear/colorless in appearance with glucose = 165 mg/dL, protein = 45 mg/dL, RBC = 10 cells/mm^3, and WBC = 5 cells/mm^3, making meningitis less likely.

QUESTIONS

1. GR is admitted and repeat blood cultures are ordered for 48 hours from the previous sets drawn in the ED. With the diagnosis of MSSA bloodstream infection, what is the most optimal change in the antimicrobial regimen for this patient at this time?
   A. Discontinue ceftriaxone, ampicillin, and dexamethasone; continue vancomycin
   B. Discontinue vancomycin, ampicillin, and dexamethasone; continue ceftriaxone
   C. Discontinue vancomycin, ceftriaxone, ampicillin, and dexamethasone; start cefazolin
   D. Discontinue vancomycin, ceftriaxone, ampicillin, and dexamethasone; start penicillin G

2. The medical intern asks if transesophageal echocardiography (TEE) is warranted in the additional workup since the patient has a prosthetic valve in the setting of MSSA bacteremia. Which of the following is true regarding TEE for this patient? A TEE is:
   A. Recommended because this patient has a prosthetic valve
   B. Not recommended because there is no evidence of endocardial involvement
   C. Not recommended because the patient already meets pathologic criteria for definitive infective endocarditis
   D. Not recommended since the TTE showed no signs of vegetation and TTE is more sensitive than TEE in the detection of intracardiac vegetations

3. A TEE is done the following morning which showed some mild mitral and tricuspid valve regurgitation as well as a 1.5 × 0.4 cm linear echo density on her prosthetic aortic valve, consistent with a vegetation. The patient is diagnosed with MSSA prosthetic aortic valve endocarditis. Cardiothoracic surgery is consulted to determine surgical management. Which of the following clinical or echocardiographic features suggest(s) the need for potential surgery? Select all that apply.
   A. Perivalvular abscess
   B. Heart failure unresponsive to medical therapy

C. A vegetation of any size on the anterior mitral leaflet

D. An embolic event during the first two weeks of antimicrobial therapy

4. Which of the following is/are true regarding *Staphylococcus aureus* infective endocarditis (IE)? Select all that apply.

A. *S. aureus* is the most common causative organism of IE in adults

B. Mortality rates associated with *S. aureus* IE range from 20% to 45%

C. Blood cultures should be repeated to confirm if this is a contaminant or a true pathogen

D. All of the above are true

5. Repeat blood cultures from hospital day (HD) 2 and HD 4 are still positive for MSSA. The team obtains an Infectious Diseases (ID) consult and is specifically wondering about the addition of gentamicin given the diagnosis of endocarditis. Which of the following is true regarding the use of gentamicin in IE?

A. Gentamicin should be added for all *S. aureus* IE, both native valve IE (NVE) and prosthetic valve IE (PVE)

B. Gentamicin is no longer indicated in the treatment of IE because risk of acute kidney injury is too high

C. If gentamicin is indicated, it should be added for the first two weeks of the IE regimen

D. If gentamicin is indicated, dosing is the same as treatment dosing of gram-negative infections

6. Gentamicin 1 mg/kg IV q8h (synergy dosing) is added by ID. On HD 6, the patient reports new headaches and is progressively more confused and somnolent. An MRI of the brain was obtained that showed several small cortical ischemic lesions concerning for septic emboli. What is the most optimal therapy for this patient in addition to continuing gentamicin?

A. Continue cefazolin

B. Change cefazolin to nafcillin

C. Change cefazolin to ceftriaxone

D. Change cefazolin to vancomycin

7. It is now HD 11 and the last set of repeat blood cultures show no growth for 4 days. The ID consult note says to add rifampin. Which of the following is true regarding the use of rifampin in IE?

A. Rifampin is only recommended for the first two weeks of IE treatment

B. It is too late to add rifampin because it should have been started on day 1 of therapy

C. Rifampin therapy is benign with minimal side effects

D. A drug interaction check should routinely be performed when adding rifampin

8. What is the appropriate duration of treatment for PVE caused by MSSA?

A. At least 4 weeks from first negative blood culture or surgical source control, whichever occurs first

B. At least 4 weeks from first negative blood culture or surgical source control, whichever occurs last

C. At least 6 weeks from first negative blood culture or surgical source control, whichever occurs first

D. At least 6 weeks from first negative blood culture or surgical source control, whichever occurs last

9. In applying the modified Duke IE criteria to this patient in retrospect, how did this patient meet the criteria for IE?

A. Two major criteria

B. One definitive histologic criteria

C. Five minor criteria

D. Without culturing the vegetation, this patient did not technically meet the Duke IE criteria

ANSWERS

1. **Explanation:** The correct answer is C. Antistaphylococcal beta-lactams (eg, cefazolin, nafcillin, oxacillin) are the treatment of choice for MSSA infections and patients should be switched as early as possible to one of these agents once MSSA has been identified as the causative agent in bacteremia (answers A and B are incorrect). Although vancomycin does provide coverage of MSSA, antistaphylococcal beta-lactams are considered superior to vancomycin, and early transition to definitive therapy with one of these agents is associated with significantly lower treatment failure, shorter time to bacteremia clearance, and most importantly, lower mortality. The majority of staphylococci (~85%) are resistant to penicillin. Because current methods for detecting penicillin susceptibility have questionable reliability and may miss more than a one-third of beta-lactamase-producing *S. aureus*, penicillin should not be used to treat *S. aureus* (answer D is incorrect).[1-4]

2. **Explanation:** The correct answer is A. Patients with infective endocarditis (IE) can present with highly variable and nonspecific symptoms making the initial differential diagnosis very broad. Echocardiography should be performed when IE is a reasonable diagnosis. TEE has been shown to be much more sensitive than TTE in the detection of intracardiac vegetations, though TTE is generally performed first if IE is suspected given the noninvasive nature of the test and is also more sensitive in detecting right-sided vegetations. However, for patients in whom there is high clinical suspicion or risk, or those where patient-specific factors prohibit an optimal echocardiographic window, a TEE should be performed first or as soon as possible after TTE since the latter cannot definitively rule out IE or potential complications (answer D is incorrect). TEE is recommended in patients with prosthetic valves, patients classified as "possible IE" by clinical criteria, or patients with complicated IE (eg, perivalvular abscess). TTE may be considered sufficient if negative in patients with low clinical suspicion for IE or if the TTE shows vegetations, the likelihood of complications is low, and obtaining a TEE will not subsequently alter management. Furthermore, repeat TEE in 7 to 10 days is warranted if there is high clinical suspicion of IE and the initial TEE results are negative. Answer B is incorrect because this patient requires further imaging to

determine if there is endocardial involvement. Answer C is incorrect because pathologic criteria require culture or histological examination of an intracardiac specimen.[4,5]

3. **Explanation:** The correct answers are A, B, and D. Several features may indicate the need for potential surgery, including both clinical and prognostic factors. Indication for surgery also depends on consideration of whether the patient has prosthetic valve (PVE) vs. native valve (NVE) IE and left- vs. right-sided IE. Generally, echocardiographic characteristics that suggest the need for surgery can be divided into three main categories: vegetation characteristics, valvular dysfunction, and perivalvular extension. Answer C is not correct as typically the greatest risk of embolic complications (and thus indication for surgery) occurs when mitral leaflet vegetations are larger than 1 cm in diameter. Additional vegetation characteristics that suggest the need for surgical intervention include an increase in vegetation size despite appropriate antimicrobial therapy, persistent vegetation after systemic embolization, or one or more embolic events during first two weeks of antimicrobial therapy (answer D). Valvular dysfunction includes acute aortic or mitral insufficiency with signs of ventricular failure, valve perforation or rupture, and heart failure unresponsive to medical therapy (answer B). Perivalvular extension includes a large abscess or extension of abscess despite appropriate medical management, new heart bock, or valvular dehiscence, rupture, or fistula (answer A). Additionally, many other clinical considerations may also drive the indication for surgery such as microbiologic factors (eg, persistent bacteremia or IE caused by fungal or highly resistant organisms) or complicated right-sided IE.[2]

4. **Explanation:** The correct answers are A and B. Staphylococci and streptococci account for 80% to 90% of IE when an identification is made. Streptococci, particularly the viridans group streptococci, are still the predominant pathogens in the developing world. However, staphylococci have assumed the role of the primary etiologic agent in the industrialized world, which is thought to be resultant of increased health care contact/exposure as a risk factor for *S. aureus* bacteremia. Of further concern is the significant morbidity and mortality associated with *S. aureus* bacteremia and IE. The primary foci of infection factors into the overall mortality rate of *S. aureus* bacteremia (SAB), but *S. aureus* IE–associated bacteremia are among the highest mortality rates, ranging from 20% to 45%. Mortality rates are typically higher in non-intravenous drug use (IVDU)–associated IE (primarily left-sided) compared to IVDU-associated IE (primarily right-sided). Answer C is incorrect because *S. aureus* should never be considered a contaminant when isolated in the blood, especially given the presence of prosthetic heart valve.[5-7]

5. **Explanation:** The correct answer is C. The addition of gentamicin is only indicated in *S. aureus* IE when there is a prosthetic valve or other prosthetic material is present (answers A and B are incorrect). The addition of

gentamicin was previously considered in select cases of NVE, but growing evidence suggests that outside of the presence of prosthetic valve/material, the risks of adding gentamicin outweigh the benefits. Gentamicin dosed for synergy should be added for the first 2 weeks of therapy provided high-level gentamicin resistance is not detected. For prosthetic valve endocarditis caused by *S. aureus,* gentamicin dosing is recommended to be 3 mg/kg/24h in 2 to 3 equally divided doses with target peaks of 3 to 4 mcg/mL and target troughs of <1 mcg/mL (answer D is incorrect). Doses should be adjusted for changes in renal function and based on therapeutic drug monitoring results.[2]

6. **Explanation:** The correct answer is B. An antistaphylococcal beta-lactam is still treatment of choice in the setting of IE with associated embolic complications (answers C and D are incorrect). Nafcillin is recommended over cefazolin and oxacillin in cases of IE complicated by septic cerebral emboli or brain abscess, owing to its more consistent blood–brain barrier penetration and greater level of evidence (answer A is incorrect). The IE guidelines also prefer nafcillin and oxacillin over cefazolin because cefazolin may be more susceptible to type A beta-lactamase-mediated hydrolysis than nafcillin, particularly in high-inoculum infections. However, clinical data to substantiate this "inoculum effect" are lacking and many clinicians may still choose to use cefazolin for tolerability and cost reasons.[2,8]

7. **Explanation:** The correct answer is D. Rifampin is used to help with sterilization of the prosthetic material and should be considered for the entire course of therapy (answer A is incorrect). However, rifampin resistance often develops rapidly if used alone or in high-inoculum infections, thus many experts recommend waiting to add rifampin until blood cultures are clear to prevent treatment-emergent rifampin resistance (answer B is incorrect). Adverse effects of rifampin include GI upset and hepatotoxicity, though typically elevations in LFTs are transient and serious hepatotoxicity is limited to patients with underlying liver injury or on concomitant hepatotoxic drugs. More notably, patients and providers should be counseled that rifampin will turn body fluids a red-orange color, including urine, tears, sweat, and even contact lenses (answer C is incorrect). Drug interactions with rifampin can be significant and are another important consideration. Rifampin is a potent inducer of CYP450 enzymes (especially CYP3A4) and most often results in decreased concentrations of drugs that are CYP450 substrates. It is important to note that enzyme induction requires upregulation or production of additional enzyme, thus the onset of drug interactions may not be immediate.[2]

8. **Explanation:** The correct answer is D. Treatment of IE is typically prolonged because of the high bacterial inoculum within vegetations, and duration is highly pathogen-specific. Other key factors that impact treatment duration include the type of valve present (NVE vs. PVE), the location of the infection (left-sided vs. right-sided), and whether the case is considered complicated or uncomplicated. In general, most

S. aureus IE should be treated for 6 weeks, with durations extended beyond 6 weeks for cases involving prosthetic valves or other complicating factors such as perivalvular abscesses. An exception may be made for uncomplicated right-sided MSSA NVE, in which treatment may be as short as 2 weeks. It is beyond the scope of this chapter to cover all commonly encountered organisms/scenarios in IE, and the authors encourage referencing the guidelines for full treatment recommendations.[2] One important summary note in managing IE: Numerous studies have shown that adherence to quality-of-care indicators (QCIs) in SAB is associated with better outcomes and reduced mortality, particularly when implemented as a bundled approach. The following QCIs should be considered standard of care in SAB: early removal of infectious foci (source control), follow-up blood cultures to assess clearance of SAB, early definitive therapy for MSSA, echocardiography, and *appropriate* treatment duration according to the complexity of the infection and/or host.[9]

9. **Explanation:** The correct answer is A. In order to meet the Duke IE criteria for definitive diagnosis of IE, a patient must have one of the following: a positive histologic result, two major criteria, five minor criteria, or one major and three minor criteria (answers B, C, and D are incorrect). The two major criteria met in this patient are supportive laboratory evidence indicated by positive blood cultures with an organism commonly associated with IE (*S. aureus*) and a positive echocardiogram (eg, vegetation by TEE). The full compilation of all modified Duke criteria is a valuable tool to review in full.[2,10]

REFERENCES

1. Richter SS, Doern GV, Heilmann KP, et al. Detection and prevalence of penicillin susceptible *Staphylococcus aureus* in the United States in 2013. *J Clin Microbiol.* 2016;54:812-814.

2. Baddour LM, Wilson WR, Bayer AS, et al. Infective endocarditis in adults: diagnosis, antimicrobial therapy, and management of complications: a scientific statement for healthcare professionals from the American Heart Association. *Circulation.* 2015;132:1435-1486.

3. Stryjewski ME, Szczech LA, Benjamin DK, et al. Use of vancomycin or first-generation cephalosporins for the treatment of hemodialysis-dependent patients with methicillin-susceptible *Staphylococcus aureus* bacteremia. *Clin Infect Dis.* 2007;44(2):190-196.

4. Siegman-Igra Y, Reich P, Orni-Wasserlauf R, Schwartz D, Giladi M. The role of vancomycin in the persistence or recurrence of *Staphylococcus aureus* bacteraemia. *Scand J Infect Dis.* 2005;37(8):572-578.

5. Fowler VG, Scheld WM, Bayer AS. Endocarditis and intravascular infections. In: Bennett JE, Dolin R, Blaser MJ, eds. *Principles and Practice of Infectious Diseases.* Philadelphia, PA: Saunders; 2015:990-1028e.11.

6. Que Y, Moreillon P. *Staphylococcus aureus* (including staphylococcal toxic shock syndrome). In: Bennett JE, Dolin R, Blaser MJ, eds. *Principles and Practice of Infectious Diseases.* Philadelphia, PA: Saunders; 2015:2237-2271e.9.

7. van Hal SJ, Jensen SO, Vaska. Predictors of mortality in *Staphylococcus aureus* bacteremia. *Clin Micro Rev.* 2012;25(2):362-386.

8. Schweizer ML, Furuno JP, Harris AD, et al. Comparative effectiveness of nafcillin or cefazolin versus vancomycin in methicillin-susceptible *Staphylococcus aureus* bacteremia. *BMC Infect Dis.* 2011;11:279.

9. López-Cortés LE, Del Toro MD, Gálvez-Acebal J, et al. Impact of an evidence-based bundle intervention in the quality-of-care management and outcome of *Staphylococcus aureus* bacteremia. *Clin Infect Dis.* 2013;57(9):1225-1233.

10. Li JS, Sexton DJ, Mick N, et al. Proposed modification to the Duke criteria for the diagnosis of infective endocarditis. *Clin Infect Dis.* 2000;30:633-638.

12 Sepsis

Emily L. Heil

PATIENT PRESENTATION

Chief Complaint
Unable to obtain due to clinical status

History of Present Illness
JG is a 72-year-old woman who was brought to the emergency department by her daughter when she noticed the patient was more confused than her baseline and was found to have a high fever with rigors. The daughter notes that the patient had complained of fatigue and back/abdominal pain accompanied by nausea and vomiting 4 days prior to presentation. JG developed respiratory distress in the emergency department and required intubation.

Past Medical History
Depression, hypertension, chronic kidney disease (baseline SCr 1.9 mg/dL), coronary artery disease—stable angina

Family History
Father passed away at age 80 from a stroke; mother had type 2 diabetes and passed secondary to breast cancer.

Social History
Widowed, lives with her daughter's family. Drinks alcohol occasionally, never smoker

Allergies
Penicillin (rash)

Home Medications
Escitalopram 10 mg PO daily
Amlodipine 10 mg PO daily
Labetalol 600 mg PO q8h
Lisinopril 40 mg PO daily
Nitroglycerin 0.4 mg sublingual PRN chest pain

Physical Exam

▶ Vital Signs
Temp 39.4°C; BP 86/50 mm Hg; MAP 62; HR 123; RR 24 breaths per minute; O_2 sat 90% on 50% FiO_2, qSOFA = 3, Wt 68 kg, Ht 5′ 4″

▶ General
Responsive, intubated, appears well nourished

▶ HEENT
Dry mucous membranes, neck supple, oropharynx clear. Endotracheal tube and nasogastric tube in place

▶ Respiratory
Respirations are unlabored and ventilator dependent. Decreased breath sounds in bilateral bases. No rales

▶ Cardiovascular
Tachycardic, normal S1-S2, regular rate and rhythm. No murmur, rubs, or gallops

▶ Abdominal
Soft, tender, non-distended, positive bowel sounds in all quadrants

▶ Genitourinary
Foley catheter in place. Moderate suprapubic tenderness

▶ Skin/Extremities
Dry, no rash. No peripheral edema

▶ Neurology
Pupils equal and reactive, alert and oriented ×2

Laboratory Findings

Na: 136 mEq/L	Hgb: 9.5 g/dL	Ca: 7.2 mg/L
K: 4.9 mEq/L	Hct: 28%	Mg: 2.0 mg/L
Cl: 100 mEq/L	Plt: 90	Phos: 5.5 mEq/L
CO_2: 11 mEq/L	WBC: 21.2×10^9/L	AST: 26 IU/L
BUN: 29 mg/dL	PT: 15.9 sec	ALT: 24 IU/L
SCr: 3.0 mg/dL	INR: 1.2	T bili: 2.0 mg/dL
Glu: 140 mg/dL	PTT: 62 sec	Alk Phos: 78 IU/L
	Lactate: 4.8 mmol/L	

ABG: 7.17/30/80/11, prior to intubation
Urine output: 40 mL in 4 hours
Urinalysis:

Appearance	Cloudy
Color	Yellow
pH	6.5
Specific gravity	1.0005
Glucose	Negative
Ketones	Negative

Leukocyte esterase	+3
Nitrites	+1
WBC/hpf	>50
RBC/hpf	0-2
Bacteria	Large
Epithelial cells	Negative

Urine and blood cultures pending

QUESTIONS

1. Based on the information provided, which of the following is the most appropriate classification of JG's condition?
   A. Sepsis
   B. Severe sepsis
   C. Septic shock
   D. Uncomplicated urinary tract infection

2. Which of the following are included in the qSOFA score for identifying high-risk patients for in-hospital mortality with suspected sepsis?
   A. Heart rate >90 bpm with vasopressor therapy
   B. Alteration of mental status
   C. Mean arterial pressure ≥65 mm Hg with vasopressor therapy
   D. Increased serum creatinine of 0.5 mg/dL from baseline or 50% increase

3. All of the following interventions should be provided to JG within her first hour of presentation according to the Surviving Sepsis Campaign 2018, *except*:
   A. Obtain blood cultures prior to administration of antibiotics
   B. Administer 30 mL/kg of crystalloid fluids for hypotension or lactate ≥4 mmol/L
   C. Administer broad-spectrum antibiotics within 1 hour of identification of sepsis
   D. Administer 30 mL/kg of 5% albumin

4. Which empiric antimicrobial therapy is most appropriate to start for JG at this time?
   A. Ceftriaxone
   B. Vancomycin + Ceftriaxone
   C. Vancomycin + Cefepime
   D. Vancomycin

5. Which of the following dosing strategies would best optimize the pharmacokinetic/pharmacodynamic principles and specific drug properties for JG's antibiotic regimen?
   A. Dosing vancomycin to achieve a trough of 5 to 10 mg/L
   B. Dosing vancomycin to achieve a trough of 20 to 25 mg/L
   C. Administering the cefepime as an extended infusion after the first dose
   D. Doubling the dose of cefepime and administering it less frequently

6. Twenty-four hours after her presentation, JG's cultures return with gram-negative rods in both her blood and urine cultures. What would be the most appropriate change to her antibiotic therapy?
   A. No changes should be made to her antibiotic therapy until full species identification and susceptibilities have been reported from the microbiology laboratory
   B. Discontinue her vancomycin and continue cefepime monotherapy
   C. Discontinue her vancomycin and cefepime; start ceftriaxone
   D. Add empiric metronidazole for coverage of gram-negative anaerobes

7. Which of the following statements regarding duration of antibiotic therapy for JG is true?
   A. All patients with septic shock should receive at least 7 days of antibiotic therapy
   B. Duration of antibiotic therapy should be chosen based on the identified source of infection
   C. Antibiotics should be discontinued after the patient's SOFA score decreases to <2
   D. Antibiotics should be given for infection prophylaxis if an alternate explanation for the shock is identified

ANSWERS

1. **Explanation:** The correct answer is C: Septic shock. Sepsis is life-threatening organ dysfunction caused by a dysregulated host response to infection.[1] The systemic inflammatory response syndrome (SIRS) criteria are no longer considered part of the definition of sepsis due to inadequate sensitivity and specificity. Instead, sepsis is defined as a suspected or documented infection with either a "quick" Sequential Organ Failure Assessment (SOFA) score of at least 2 or an acute increase of ≥2 points on the full SOFA score. Severe sepsis was an old definition from a 1991 consensus conference that was sepsis complicated by organ dysfunction. This definition was sunset with the 2016 Sepsis-3 Consensus Definitions. Septic shock is a subset of sepsis where underlying circulatory and cellular abnormalities are profound enough that the patient is at substantially increased risk of mortality. Patients with septic shock meet the definition for sepsis and have hypotension requiring vasopressor therapy to maintain a MAP ≥65 mm Hg and having a serum lactate level greater than 2 mmol/L after adequate fluid resuscitation.[1] While we do not have information on current medications for JG, we do know that her MAP is <65 mm Hg and her lactate is >2 mmol/L indicating that she has septic shock.

2. **Explanation:** The correct answer is B. The Quick Sequential Organ Failure Assessment (qSOFA) criteria are alteration in mental status, systolic blood pressure ≤100 mm Hg or respiratory rate ≥22 breaths/min. Patients with a score of 2 to 3 are at a 3–14-fold increase for in-hospital mortality. The tool was introduced by the Sepsis-3 task force as a rapid bedside clinical score that could be used to identify patients with a suspected infection at a greater risk

for mortality. The score is meant to replace the systemic inflammatory response syndrome (SIRS) criteria that were previously used to identify sepsis as they are less sensitive and specific.[1,2]

3. **Explanation:** The correct answer is D. The Surviving Sepsis Campaign bundle was updated in 2018 to a single "hour-1 bundle" of resuscitation and management recommendations that should be completed within the first hour of identification of sepsis or septic shock. The bundle elements include measuring a lactate level, obtaining blood cultures *prior* to the administration of antibiotics, administering broad-spectrum antibiotics, beginning rapid resuscitation by administering 30 mL/kg of crystalloid (eg, normal saline, lactated ringers) for hypotension or lactate ≥4 mmol/L and to apply vasopressors if patients remain hypotensive during or after fluid resuscitation to maintain a MAP ≥65 mm Hg.[3] Administration of colloids such as albumin is not recommended as part of the bundle due to an absence of data supporting a clear benefit to colloids compared to crystalloids for resuscitation in sepsis.

4. **Explanation:** The correct answer is C. One of the most important interventions in the management of a patient with septic shock is prompt initiation of broad-spectrum antibiotics with coverage of gram-positive and gram-negative organisms. Antibiotics should ideally be given with 1 hour of the patient's presentation with septic shock but after appropriate cultures have been obtained.[3] Failure to promptly initiate appropriate antibiotic therapy is associated with increased morbidity and mortality in patients with sepsis and septic shock.[4] Antibiotic selection should be chosen based upon patient-specific factors such as the suspected site of infection, chronic organ failures, recent infections or known colonization with other organisms, and allergies. Other factors to consider are the prevalence of certain pathogens such as methicillin-resistant *Staphylococcus aureus* (MRSA) within the community and the hospital, which can be found in local antibiograms.[4] Typically, therapy involved an agent with MRSA coverage plus an anti-pseudomonal beta-lactam such as a broad-spectrum carbapenem (eg, meropenem, imipenem/cilastatin), a higher-generation cephalosporin (eg, ceftazidime or cefepime), or an extended-range penicillin/beta-lactamase inhibitor combination (eg, piperacillin/tazobactam). Based on JG's symptoms, it is likely that she has sepsis from a urinary source so the most likely pathogens would be gram-negative bacteria; however, given the severity of her presentation, she should be provided with broad-spectrum coverage of both gram-positive and gram-negative organisms until her cultures return. As JG has a reported allergy to penicillins, with limited history on the reaction and timeline, use of the fourth-generation cephalosporin cefepime is unlikely to result in an allergic reaction due to low rates of cross-reactivity and can be used for broad-spectrum coverage including *Pseudomonas aeruginosa*.[5] Often in empiric treatment of sepsis, vancomycin

is added to provide broad-spectrum gram-positive coverage including MRSA; however, vancomycin alone would be inappropriate as it only provides gram-positive coverage. The options of ceftriaxone monotherapy or vancomycin plus ceftriaxone alone are inadequate as ceftriaxone does not provide coverage of *P. aeruginosa*. Once JG's cultures return, her antibiotic therapy should be promptly narrowed to eliminate any unnecessary coverage.

5. **Explanation:** The correct answer is C. Early optimization of antimicrobial dosing is important to improve outcomes in patients with severe infections, particularly as critically patients often have altered pharmacokinetics. Vancomycin's efficacy is best described by the area under the concentration-time curve to minimum inhibitory concentration ratio (AUC:MIC). Trough concentrations are typically used as a surrogate marker with troughs of 15 to 20 mg/L used for serious infections. A trough concentration target of 5 to 10 mg/L is too low and risks the development of resistance, whereas a trough concentration >20 mg/L puts the patient at increased risk of vancomycin-associated nephrotoxicity.[6] For beta-lactams, the pharmacokinetic/pharmacodynamics target is maximizing time that the plasma concentration of the drug is above the pathogen MIC relative to the dosing interval. The best way to do this is to extend the infusion of the drug for several hours. The first dose should be given as a bolus to rapidly achieve therapeutic blood levels with the infusion time extended for subsequent doses only. If extended infusions cannot be used due to things such as insufficient line access, increasing the frequency of dosing is a simple way to increase time above MIC.[4]

6. **Explanation:** The correct answer is B. Due to the increasing frequency of antibiotic resistance worldwide, it is important to avoid unnecessary use of broad-spectrum antibiotics whenever possible. Given the high mortality associated with sepsis and septic shock, it is appropriate to provide empiric broad-spectrum therapy until a causative organism and its susceptibilities are defined.[4] However, attempts to eliminate coverage that is no longer needed and to de-escalate broad-spectrum agents to more narrow-spectrum agents tailored toward the patient's cultures are an important antimicrobial stewardship initiative. At this point, we know that JG's cultures have gram-negative organisms, so discontinuing her broad-spectrum gram-positive coverage that was provided by vancomycin is appropriate. Since we do not have further identification of the organism, it would not be appropriate to de-escalate to ceftriaxone from cefepime, as anti-pseudomonal coverage is still warranted. Adding metronidazole for gram-negative anaerobic coverage is not indicated at this time as these organisms would be unlikely causative agents for a urinary source of infection.

7. **Explanation:** The correct answer is B. Most infections can be adequately treated with a 7-day course of antimicrobial therapy; however, some infections have data for shorter courses such as intra-abdominal sepsis with source control, and some require much longer courses such as complicated

S. aureus bacteremia. Therefore, the primary driver for duration of therapy in patients with septic shock should be based on the underlying source of infection identified. For JG, since it has been determined that she had sepsis from a urinary source, her duration of therapy would be guided by the therapeutic guidelines for complicated urinary tract infections. While resolution of symptoms is an important factor in determining if it is appropriate to stop a patient's antibiotics, use of the SOFA score to dictate duration is not appropriate. Additionally, antibiotics should be promptly discontinued when patients have severe inflammatory states of non-infectious origin, and not be used for prophylaxis.[4]

REFERENCES

1. Singer M, Deutschman CS, Seymour CW, et al. The Third International Consensus Definitions for Sepsis and Septic Shock (Sepsis-3). *JAMA*. 2016;315:801-810.

2. Seymour CW, Liu VK, Iwashyna TJ, et al. Assessment of clinical criteria for sepsis for the Third International Consensus Definitions for Sepsis and Septic Shock (Sepsis-3). *JAMA*. 2016;315:762-774.

3. Levy M, Evans LE, Rhodes A. The surviving sepsis campaign bundle: 2018 update. *Crit Care Med*. 2018;46:997-1000.

4. Rhodes A, Evans LE, Alhazzani W, et al. Surviving sepsis campaign: International Guidelines for Management of Sepsis and Septic Shock: 2016. *Crit Care Med*. 2017;45:486-552.

5. Campagna JD, Bond MC, Schabelman E, Hayes BD. The use of cephalosporins in penicillin-allergic patients: a literature review. *J Emerg Med*. 2012;42:612-620.

6. Rybak MJ, Lomaestro BM, Rotschafer JC, et al. Vancomycin therapeutic guidelines: a summary of consensus recommendations from the Infectious Diseases Society of America, the American Society of Health-System Pharmacists, and the Society of Infectious Diseases Pharmacists. *Clin Infect Dis*. 2009;49:325-327.

13 Human Immunodeficiency Virus and Opportunistic Infections

Elizabeth Sherman

PATIENT PRESENTATION

Chief Complaint

"I'm here for my follow-up visit to start HIV treatment and I'm concerned about these white spots in my mouth. This is the first time I have had them; they don't go away. I tried to scrape them off and they just come back."

History of Present Illness

AS is a 25-year-old woman who comes to the family health clinic for her routine HIV care, where she had deferred starting antiretroviral therapy because she "felt fine" and because she was "not sure those drugs work anyway." Six weeks ago, while on an extended family vacation she was admitted to the hospital with *Pneumocystis jirovecii* pneumonia. Upon discharge, she saw a physician friend of the family who convinced her to start an antiretroviral regimen. Today the patient complains of white, non-painful, plaques inside her mouth and on her tongue for the past two weeks consistent with oropharyngeal candidiasis.

Past Medical History

HIV diagnosed 2 years ago; risk factor: heterosexual contact
Pneumocystis pneumonia diagnosed 6 weeks ago
History of peptic ulcer 4 years ago, treated with antibiotic therapy and maintained on PPI

Surgical History

None

Family History

Father has hypertension and hyperlipidemia; mother has breast cancer and hyperlipidemia

Social History

Works as a cashier at a grocery store. Single, sexually active with a monogamous male partner, does not regularly use contraception, lives alone. Never smoked, drinks occasionally (2 to 4 drinks per week on the weekend).

Allergies

Sulfa (history of trimethoprim/sulfamethoxazole causing Stevens–Johnson syndrome)

Medications

Atovaquone 1500 mg (10 mL) PO daily
Omeprazole 20 mg PO daily

Physical Examination

▶ *Vital Signs*

Temp 98.9°F, P 87 beats per minute, RR 13 breaths per minute, BP 125/76 mm Hg, Ht 5′9″, Wt 72 kg

▶ *General*

Pleasant, pale-looking female in no acute distress

▶ *HEENT*

Normocephalic, atraumatic, PERRLA, EOMI, visible white plaques on the buccal area and tongue (no plaques seen in throat), poor dentition, L neck lymph node 0.8 cm in diameter

▶ *Pulmonary*

Effort normal and breath sounds normal

▶ *Cardiovascular*

Normal rate, regular rhythm, and normal heart sounds

▶ **Abdomen**

Soft, non-distended, non-tender, bowel sounds normal

▶ **Genitourinary**

Deferred

▶ **Neurology**

A&O ×3

▶ **Extremities**

Normal

Laboratory Findings

Na = 141 mEq/L   Hgb = 12 g/dL   Ca = 9.3 mg/dL

K = 4.2 mEq/L   Hct = 39% PO_4 = 3.8 mEq/L

Cl = 103 mEq/L   Plt = 206 ×10^3/mm^3 AST = 20 IU/L

CO_2 = 27 mEq/L   WBC = 7.3 ×10^3 mm^3 ALT = 31 IU/L

BUN = 12 mg/dL   T Bili =
                                       0.7 mg/dL

SCr = 1.1 mg/dL   Alk Phos =
                                       76 IU/L

Glu = 95 mg/dL

CD4+ 78 cells/mm^3 (6 weeks ago during hospitalization)
HIV RNA 123,000 copies/mL (6 weeks ago during hospitalization)
CD4+ 68 cells/mm^3 (today)
HIV RNA 127,000 copies/mL (today)
Toxoplasmosis IgG (+)
HLA-B*5701 (+)

QUESTIONS

1. Which information (signs, symptoms, laboratory values) from AS's case indicates an AIDS diagnosis?
   A. Lymphadenopathy
   B. Oral candidiasis
   C. HIV RNA above 100,000 copies/mL
   D. CD4 + below 200 cells/mm^3

2. What should AS be told regarding the need for antiretroviral therapy?
   A. Therapy is recommended for all persons with HIV infection
   B. Therapy is recommended only for persons who have a documented decline in CD4+ of at least 100 cells/mm^3
   C. Therapy can be considered but is not necessarily recommended
   D. Therapy is recommended only for persons who have an HIV RNA above 30,000 copies/mL

3. For which opportunistic infection does AS require primary prophylaxis?
   A. *Toxoplasma gondii* encephalitis
   B. *Mycobacterium avium* complex disease
   C. *Pneumocystis jirovecii* pneumonia
   D. Oral candidiasis

4. Which of the following describes a recommended initial antiretroviral regimen for most people with HIV that should be recommended to AS?
   A. 1 integrase strand transfer inhibitor + 2 nucleos(t)ide reverse transcriptase inhibitors
   B. 1 boosted protease inhibitor + 2 nucleos(t)ide reverse transcriptase inhibitors
   C. 1 non-nucleoside reverse transcriptase inhibitor + 2 nucleos(t)ide reverse transcriptase inhibitors
   D. 1 entry inhibitor + 2 nucleos(t)ide reverse transcriptase inhibitors

5. Which one of the following is considered a recommended initial regimen for most people with HIV and represents the best regimen for AS?
   A. Rilpivirine-tenofovir disoproxil fumarate-emtricitabine
   B. Darunavir-cobicistat plus abacavir-lamivudine
   C. Elvitegravir/cobicistat/tenofovir alafenamide/emtricitabine
   D. Bictegravir-tenofovir alafenamide-emtricitabine

6. After initiating antiretroviral therapy, which one of the following approaches is recommended for monitoring AS's initial response to treatment?
   A. Monitor the CD4 count monthly until greater than 500 cells/mm^3
   B. Check the HIV RNA within 2 to 4 weeks and then every 4 to 8 weeks until the HIV RNA level is below the assay's limit of detection
   C. Repeat the HIV RNA and CD4 count every 16 weeks until steady state is reached
   D. Monitor the HIV RNA every 4 weeks until below 200 copies/mL, then monitor every 12 weeks until below the assay's limit of detection

7. AS has a urine pregnancy test performed in the clinic today and it is negative. She states that her male partner uses condoms "most of the time." She inquires into using a combination oral contraceptive containing levonorgestrel and ethinyl estradiol. Which one of the following antiretroviral regimens would present the lowest risk for drug–drug interactions with this oral contraceptive?
   A. Efavirenz-tenofovir disoproxil fumarate-emtricitabine
   B. Darunavir plus ritonavir plus tenofovir disoproxil fumarate-emtricitabine
   C. Dolutegravir plus tenofovir alafenamide-emtricitabine
   D. Elvitegravir-cobicistat-tenofoviralafenamide-emtricitabine

8. Which one of the following is recommended for the initial treatment of AS's oral candidiasis infection?
   A. Liposomal amphotericin B 3 to 4 mg/kg IV daily for 21 days

B. Micafungin 150 mg IV daily for 14 days

C. Fluconazole 100 mg PO daily for 14 days

D. Itraconazole capsules 200 mg PO daily for 21 days

9. AS asks if she can stop taking atovaquone. Which of the following is one of the recommended indications for discontinuing *Pneumocystis* pneumonia secondary prophylaxis?

A. Normal chest radiograph 6 months after starting antiretroviral therapy

B. CD4+ increased from below 200 cells/mm³ to above 200 cells/mm³ for more than 3 months in response to antiretroviral therapy

C. CD4+ above 100 cells/mm³ for more than 6 weeks in response to antiretroviral therapy

D. Undetectable HIV RNA for more than 6 months in response to antiretroviral therapy, regardless of CD4+

ANSWERS

1. **Explanation:** The correct answer is D. An individual is diagnosed with AIDS when he or she has HIV and certain laboratory values, signs, or symptoms defined by the U.S. Centers for Disease Control and Prevention (CDC).[1] The CDC's definition of AIDS includes CD4+ below 200 cells/mm³, a CD4 percentage below 14% of all lymphocytes, or one or more AIDS defining conditions. AS's physical exam reveals lymphadenopathy and presumptive oral candidiasis, which are not AIDS-defining conditions. While candidiasis of the esophagus, bronchi, trachea, or lungs are AIDS-defining conditions, candidiasis of the buccal area and tongue are not (rules out answers A and B). HIV RNA values do not indicate an AIDS diagnosis (rules out answer C). Therefore, the only criterion in AS's case indicating an AIDS diagnosis is her CD4+ below 200 cells/mm³.

2. **Explanation:** The correct answer is A. According to the United States Department of Health and Human Services (DHHS) guidelines panel, antiretroviral therapy is recommended for all individuals with HIV infection, regardless of CD4 cell count or HIV RNA, to reduce morbidity and mortality associated with HIV infection and to prevent HIV transmission.[2]

3. **Explanation:** The correct answer is A. Primary prophylaxis is defined as a medication given to a patient with no prior history or diagnosis of the opportunistic infection, but who is at risk of developing the opportunistic infection. Secondary prophylaxis, also known as chronic maintenance therapy, is defined as a medication given to a patient to prevent a recurrence of a prior, successfully controlled infection. Primary prophylaxis against toxoplasmosis is indicated if the CD4+ is below 100 cells/mm³ and the patient is positive for toxoplasma IgG.[1] Because AS meets both of these criteria, she is a candidate for *Toxoplasma gondii* encephalitis primary prophylaxis. Primary prophylaxis for disseminated *Mycobacterium avium* complex disease is only indicated if CD4+ is below

50 cells/mm³ after ruling out disseminated active MAC infection and if the patient is not immediately initiating ART, is not receiving ART, or remains viremic while on ART with no options for a fully suppressive ART regimen (rules out answer B).[1] Because AS has already had *Pneumocystis jirovecii* pneumonia, she is not a candidate for primary prophylaxis, but rather she is a candidate for secondary prophylaxis (rules out answer C). Routine primary prophylaxis for oral candidiasis is not recommended (rules out answer D).[1]

4. **Explanation:** The correct answer is A. According to DHHS guidelines, the recommended initial regimen for most people with HIV is a two-drug nucleos(t)ide reverse transcriptase inhibitor (NRTI) backbone combined with an integrase strand transfer inhibitor (INSTI) anchor drug.[2] Regimens that include a boosted protease inhibitor or a non-nucleoside reverse transcriptase inhibitor are reserved only for certain clinical situations.[2] Antiretroviral regimens that include an entry inhibitor are not recommended in initial regimens for treatment-naïve patients.[2] This information was up to date as of the writing of this chapter; however, these recommendations change often. Please check for updates at aidsinfo.nih.gov.

5. **Explanation:** The correct answer is D. According to DHHS guidelines the recommended initial regimen for most people with HIV is a two-drug NRTI backbone combined with an INSTI anchor drug (rules out answers A and B which are NNRTI- and PI-based, respectively).[2] Additionally, AS's HLA-B*5701 test result was positive, indicating that she is likely to develop a hypersensitivity reaction to abacavir (rules out answer B). In this case, abacavir should not be used and a true abacavir allergy should be recorded in AS's medical chart even though she has never received the drug. Elvitegravir is an integrase inhibitor; however, due to its need for pharmacokinetic enhancement and lower genetic barrier to resistance, it is now only recommended for initial therapy in certain clinical situations (rules out answer C). The best answer choice is D, which represents a guideline-preferred regimen for most patients with HIV.

6. **Explanation:** The correct answer is B. After initiating antiretroviral therapy, the recommended laboratory monitoring approach is to recheck HIV RNA within 2 to 4 weeks (and no later than 8 weeks) and then recheck every 4 to 8 weeks until the HIV RNA level is below the limit of detection; subsequently, the HIV RNA should be rechecked every 3 to 4 months (rules out answers C and D).[2] For individuals with consistently suppressed HIV RNA levels for at least 2 years, clinicians may extend the interval for monitoring HIV RNA.[2] Additionally, although the CD4 count is a key factor in assessing the patient's overall immune status, frequent monitoring of the CD4 cell count in the initial 12 weeks after starting antiretroviral therapy does not provide meaningful information

(rules out answer A). It is recommended to check a CD4 cell count 3 months after starting antiretroviral therapy. Thereafter, the CD4 count should be monitored every 3 to 6 months for the first 2 years after starting antiretroviral therapy. For patients who have persistently undetectable HIV RNA levels and a CD4 count above 300 cells/mm³, monitoring of the CD4 cell count can be extended.

7. **Explanation:** The correct answer is C. Both estrogen and progestin are predominantly metabolized via the cytochrome P450 system and can interact with multiple antiretroviral agents. Any major alteration in levels of oral contraceptive agents can result in contraception failure and unintended pregnancy. Dolutegravir does not have any significant drug interactions with oral contraceptives, and thus provides a safe option for coadministration with oral contraceptives.[2] Preliminary data suggest an increased risk of neural tube defects in infants born to women who were receiving dolutegravir at the time of conception.[2] For those using effective contraception, such as the hormonal contraceptive described above, a dolutegravir-based regimen can be considered. Dolutegravir should not be prescribed to women who are pregnant and within 12 weeks post-conception; or who are of childbearing potential and planning to become pregnant; or who are of childbearing potential, sexually active, and not using effective contraception.[2] Although efavirenz does not significantly alter ethinyl estradiol plasma concentrations, it decreases levonorgestrel levels by 83%; if efavirenz is used with an oral hormonal contraceptive, the recommendation is to use alternative or additional contraceptive methods (rules out answer A).[2] Ritonavir-boosted protease inhibitor regimens cause a moderate decrease in plasma levels of ethinyl estradiol and norethindrone, warranting the recommendation to consider using alternative or additional contraceptive methods or an alternative antiretroviral regimen (rules out answer B).[2] The effects of cobicistat on hormonal contraceptives have not been well studied and experts recommend using alternative methods of contraception if a cobicistat-containing regimen is used (rules out answer D).[2]

8. **Explanation:** The correct answer is C. Oral fluconazole for 7 to 14 days is considered the drug of choice to treat oropharyngeal candidiasis.[1] Intravenous antifungal agents are not warranted for oropharyngeal candidiasis, although they are considered alternative therapy to fluconazole for the treatment of more severe candida infections such as esophageal candidiasis (rules out answers A and B).[1] Itraconazole capsules are less effective than fluconazole because of their more variable absorption and are associated with more drug–drug interactions than fluconazole (rules out answer D).[1] Additionally, itraconazole absorption is dependent on gastric acidity and, therefore, the patient's use of a proton pump inhibitor would interact with itraconazole capsules.

9. **Explanation:** The correct answer is B. All patients diagnosed with *Pneumocystis* pneumonia should receive chronic maintenance therapy (secondary prophylaxis) after completing the initial 21-day treatment course.[1] The Opportunistic Infections Guidelines recommend discontinuation of secondary prophylaxis for *Pneumocystis* pneumonia if a patient has responded to antiretroviral therapy with a sustained increase in CD4+ from below 200 cells/mm³ to above 200 cells/mm³ for longer than 3 months.[1] In addition, the Opportunistic Infections Guidelines note that clinicians can consider discontinuing secondary prophylaxis for *Pneumocystis* pneumonia if the patient has a CD4+ 100 to 200 cells/mm³ and the HIV RNA has remained below the limit of detection for at least 3 to 6 months.[1] Note that for *Pneumocystis* pneumonia, the criteria for discontinuing and restarting secondary prophylaxis are the same as for discontinuing and restarting primary prophylaxis.

REFERENCES

1. Panel on Opportunistic Infections in HIV-Infected Adults and Adolescents. Guidelines for the prevention and treatment of opportunistic infections in HIV-infected adults and adolescents: recommendations from the Centers for Disease Control and Prevention, the National Institutes of Health, and the HIV Medicine Association of the Infectious Diseases Society of America. Available at https://aidsinfo.nih.gov/guidelines/html/4/adult-and-adolescent-oi-prevention-and-treatment-guidelines/0. Accessed March 25, 2019.

2. Panel on Antiretroviral Guidelines for Adults and Adolescents. Guidelines for the use of antiretroviral agents in adults and adolescents living with HIV. Department of Health and Human Services. Available at https://aidsinfo.nih.gov/guidelines/html/1/adult-and-adolescent-treatment-guidelines/0. AccessedMarch 25, 2019.

14 Febrile Neutropenia

Wesley D. Kufel

PATIENT PRESENTATION

Chief Complaint

"I have a fever and chills."

History of Present Illness

JP is a 34-year-old Caucasian male who is admitted to inpatient oncology service for induction chemotherapy for a recent diagnosis of acute myeloid leukemia (AML). His induction chemotherapy regimen consists of 7 + 3 induction chemotherapy with cytarabine and daunorubicin. He was placed on neutropenic precautions, started on appropriate antimicrobial prophylaxis, and a port was placed for chemotherapy administration. Ten days after the completion of his induction chemotherapy (day 17), he spiked a fever of 38.8°C (101.8°F) and complained of chills and nausea. Details of the hospital course by day are detailed below:

Day	1	2	3	4	7	9	12	17
WBC	4.5	4.1	3.7	3.2	1.4	0.7	0.2	0.1
Comments	Daunorubicin and cytarabine started	–	Daunorubicin completed; nausea	Nausea	Cytarabine completed; nausea	Nausea	Nausea	Fever, chills, nausea (current presentation)

Past Medical History

Epilepsy, depression

Surgical History

Appendectomy (10 years ago)

Family History

Father had AML and passed away 8 years ago; mother has hypertension and epilepsy; no siblings

Social History

Married with twins (5 years old). Has never smoked and denies illicit drug use. Drinks alcohol socially. He was previously enlisted in the Navy and is currently a gym teacher at a local elementary school.

Allergies

Penicillin (reaction: rash)

Home Medications

Sertraline 1000 mg PO daily
Divalproex sodium delayed-release 1000 mg PO BID
Levetiracetam 1000 mg PO BID
Multivitamin PO daily

Inpatient Medications

Sertraline 1000 mg PO daily
Divalproex sodium delayed-release 1000 mg PO BID
Levetiracetam 1000 mg PO BID
Posaconazole delayed-release 300 mg PO BID ×1 day followed by 300 mg PO daily (day 1 start)
Valacyclovir 500 mg PO BID (day 1 start)
Levofloxacin 500 mg PO daily (day 1 start)

Review of Systems (day 17)

Positive for fever, chills, and nausea; denies vomiting, cough, diarrhea, or abdominal pain

Physical Examination (day 17)

▶ *Vital Signs*

Temp 38.8°C, P 105 bpm, RR 16 breaths per minute, BP 112/78 mm Hg, pO_2 98%, Ht 5′ 8″, Wt 74 kg

▶ *General*

Male with fatigue and in mild to moderate distress

▶ *HEENT*

PERRLA, EOMI, good dentition, no rhinorrhea or mucositis

> ### *Pulmonary*

Normal lung sounds; no wheezes, crackles, or rhonchi

> ### *Cardiovascular*

Tachycardic but regular rhythm; no murmurs, rubs, or gallops

> ### *Abdomen*

Soft, non-distended, non-tender, normal bowel sounds

> ### *Genitourinary*

Normal male genitalia, no complaints of dysuria or hematuria, prostate exam not performed

> ### *Neurology*

A & O ×3

> ### *Extremities*

Warm and dry. No erythema or induration around port on the left chest. No rashes present

Laboratory Findings (day 17)

Na = 135 mEq/L	Ca = 8.0 mg/dL	Lymphs = 81%
K = 4.0 mEq/L	Hgb = 7.8 g/dL	AST = 18 IU/L
Cl = 97 mEq/L	Hct = 23.4%	ALT = 22 IU/L
CO_2 = 25 mEq/L	Plt = 23×10^3/mm^3	T Bili = 0.8 mg/dL
BUN = 14 mg/dL	WBC = 0.1 cells/mm^3	Alk Phos = 40 IU/L
SCr = 0.8 mg/dL	PMNs = 14%	HSV IgG = positive (day 1 lab)
Glc = 84 mg/dL	Bands = 5%	CMV IgG = negative (day 1 lab)

> ### *Blood Cultures*

Periphery ×2 (pending); port catheter (pending)

> ### *Urinalysis*

0 WBC, leukocyte esterase negative, nitrite negative; urine culture not performed

> ### *Methicillin-Resistant Staphylococcus aureus (MRSA) Nasal Polymerase Chain Reaction (PCR) Screen*

Negative

> ### *Chest X-ray*

Lungs are clear

QUESTIONS

1. Which of the following is the correct absolute neutrophil count (ANC) for JP on day 17?
   A. 100/mm^3
   B. 19/mm^3
   C. 14/mm^3
   D. 5/mm^3

2. Which of the following is TRUE regarding neutropenic fever?
   A. Common signs and symptoms of infection are often absent
   B. An oral temperature of 37.8°C represents a fever
   C. Febrile neutropenia is more common in solid tumor patients compared to acute leukemia patients
   D. Chemotherapy-induced mucositis is an uncommon cause of neutropenic fever

3. Which of the following is TRUE regarding infectious pathogens in patients with neutropenic fever?
   A. Fungi are the most frequent cause of neutropenic fever
   B. Gram-positive bacterial infections are more common than gram-negative bacterial infections in neutropenic fever
   C. Infectious sources are frequently identified in febrile neutropenia cases
   D. Viruses should not be considered in the workup of neutropenic fever

4. Based on this patient's history, how should you categorize JP's neutropenic fever risk?
   A. Low risk → Treat as outpatient with oral antibiotics
   B. Low risk → Treat as outpatient with intravenous antibiotics
   C. High risk → Treat as inpatient with oral antibiotics
   D. High risk → Treat as inpatient with intravenous antibiotics

5. Which of the following antibiotics should be started for JP on day 17 in response to his fever spike?
   A. Discontinue levofloxacin prophylaxis and start ertapenem
   B. Discontinue levofloxacin prophylaxis and start piperacillin-tazobactam
   C. Discontinue levofloxacin prophylaxis and start cefepime
   D. Discontinue levofloxacin prophylaxis and start meropenem

6. Intravenous vancomycin should be added to JP's empiric antibiotic regimen.
   A. True
   B. False

7. JP was started on appropriate empiric antibacterial therapy based on the pharmacist's recommendations. Blood cultures from the port and periphery were collected prior to antibiotic administration on day 17. On day 18, both blood cultures were positive with gram-negative rods on Gram stain. On day 19, both blood cultures are growing *Pseudomonas aeruginosa* with the following susceptibility results: piperacillin-tazobactam (susceptible); ceftazidime (susceptible); cefepime (susceptible); meropenem (susceptible); ciprofloxacin (resistant); gentamicin (susceptible); tobramycin (susceptible). Which of the following would be

the MOST appropriate recommendation for management in this patient?

A. Remove the catheter/port and continue cefepime

B. Remove the catheter/port, discontinue cefepime, and start meropenem

C. Retain the catheter/port, start gentamicin lock therapy, and continue cefepime

D. Remove the catheter/port, continue cefepime, and add gentamicin

8. Empiric antifungal therapy should be considered after 4 to 7 days of appropriate empiric antibacterial therapy in high-risk neutropenic patients who continue to be febrile.

A. True

B. False

ANSWERS

1. **Explanation:** The correct answer is B. The absolute neutrophil count (ANC) determines the degree of neutropenia.[1,2] The ANC is calculated by adding the percent of polymorphonuclear cells (PMNs) (or the mature segs) to the percent of bands (immature form) and multiply this percentage by the total white blood cell (WBC) count. In this case, the total WBC count is 100 and percent PMNs or segs are 14% and the percent bands are 5%. When these values are added together, the total percentage is 19%. When the total percentage (19% or 0.19) is multiplied by the total WBC count (100), the ANC is calculated as $19/mm^3$ making option B correct. Option A represents the WBC count. Option C represents the WBC multiplied by the percent PMNs only. Option D represents the WBC multiplied by the percent bands only. The definition of neutropenia can vary between institutions, but is usually defined as an absolute neutrophil count (ANC) <1500 or $1000/mm^3$, and severe neutropenia is usually defined as an ANC <$500/mm^3$ or an ANC that is expected to decrease to <$500/mm^3$ over the next 48 hours. Profound neutropenia is typically defined as an ANC <$100/mm^3$. This patient has an ANC <$100/mm^3$, which is considered as profound neutropenia.

2. **Explanation:** The correct answer is A. Option A is correct since common signs and symptoms of infection are often absent in neutropenic fever because the magnitude of the neutrophil-mediated component of the inflammatory response may be blunted in neutropenic patients.[1,2] These patients may not have the same clinical presentation or signs and symptoms as immunocompetent patients. Fever is defined as a single oral temperature of ≥38.3°C (101.4 °F) or an oral temperature of 38°C to 38.2°C (100.4 to 100.9°F) persisting for one hour or longer. Therefore, option B does not represent a fever. Febrile neutropenia is more common in acute leukemia patients and patients with hematologic malignancies compared to patients with solid tumors. Therefore, option C is incorrect. Chemotherapy-induced mucositis is a common cause of neutropenic fever, making answer choice D incorrect.

The most common contributing factors of neutropenic fever are the direct effects of chemotherapy on mucosal barriers and the immune system as well as breeches in host defense mechanisms. Mucositis occurs when normal flora (ie, from the gastrointestinal tract) crosses mucosal membranes and translocates into the bloodstream causing infection.

3. **Explanation:** The correct answer is B. Bacteria are the most frequent infectious causes of neutropenic fever rather than fungi.[1,2] The risk for invasive fungal infections increases with the duration and severity of neutropenia, prolonged antibiotic therapy, and number or intensity of chemotherapy. Fungi are rarely identified as the cause of the first febrile episode, but rather after 1 to 2 weeks of neutropenia. This makes option A incorrect. Gram-negative bacteria were historically the most common cause of neutropenic fever, but gram-positive bacteria have become the most common pathogens. Many gram-positive bacteria are considered normal flora on the skin; however, less virulent bacteria (ie, coagulase-negative staphylococci) may become pathogenic in neutropenic patients where host immunity is compromised. Additionally, oral levofloxacin is commonly used for prophylaxis in neutropenic patients, and generally has greater activity against gram-negative bacteria compared to certain gram-positive bacteria. This makes option B correct. Unfortunately, an infectious source is often only identified in approximately 20% to 30% of febrile neutropenia cases. This makes neutropenic fever challenging for clinicians especially if the source of infection is not clearly identified. This makes option C incorrect. Viral infections are common in high-risk patients with febrile neutropenia. Human herpesviruses are among the most common viral pathogens especially in patients who are seropositive. This makes option D incorrect. In this case, JP's herpes simplex virus (HSV) IgG was positive and reactivation of latent infection is common in this scenario. Therefore, patients typically receive an antiviral (ie, valacyclovir) for HSV prophylaxis. Patients with AML who undergo induction chemotherapy are commonly given an extended-spectrum azole antifungal with mold coverage (ie, posaconazole) for prophylaxis against fungal infections as well.

4. **Explanation:** The correct answer is D. Risk assessment is needed to determine the type of empiric antibiotic therapy (oral vs intravenous), location of treatment (inpatient vs outpatient), and duration of antibiotic therapy.[1,2] High-risk patients are considered to be those with anticipated prolonged (>7 days duration) and profound neutropenia (ANC ≤$100/mm^3$) following cytotoxic chemotherapy and/or significant medical comorbidities including hypotension, pneumonia, abdominal pain, or neurologic changes. These patients should be admitted to the hospital for empiric intravenous antibiotics. Risk classification may also be calculated using the Multinational Association for Supportive Care in Cancer (MASCC) risk index

score. High-risk patients have a MASCC score <21, whereas low-risk patients have a MASCC score ≥21 and may be candidates for oral antibiotics as an outpatient. JP is considered high risk given his profound neutropenia and anticipated prolonged duration of neutropenia secondary to his chemotherapy regimen's high likelihood of neutropenic duration. Therefore, he should remain as an inpatient and receive intravenous empiric antibiotics. A MASCC score could also be used to help calculate JP's risk.

5. **Explanation:** The correct answer is C. Neutropenic fever is considered a medical emergency.[1,2] In patients that are considered high-risk, empiric intravenous (IV) antibiotic therapy should be initiated promptly within the first 60 minutes of presentation and directed against *Pseudomonas aeruginosa* after blood cultures and other cultures have been obtained if suspecting infection at specific sites (ie, urine, sputum). Anti-pseudomonal beta-lactam antibiotics are preferred over fluoroquinolones and aminoglycosides as monotherapy in neutropenic fever. Several combination antibiotic regimens have been studied as initial empiric therapy in neutropenic fever, but none have been shown to be clearly superior to others or to monotherapy antibiotic regimens. Ertapenem is a carbapenem antibiotic that does not exhibit activity against *P. aeruginosa* and should not be recommended. This makes option A incorrect. Piperacillin-tazobactam, cefepime, meropenem, and imipenem-cilastatin are all reasonable antibiotics to consider for empiric antibiotic therapy in febrile neutropenia due to their activity against *P. aeruginosa*. Higher doses of intravenous anti-pseudomonal beta-lactams are typically recommended assuming normal renal function given the severity of the infection (Table 14.1). Extended infusion or continuous infusion strategies may be implemented to optimize beta-lactam antibiotics' time-dependent pharmacodynamics. This patient has a penicillin allergy with a reaction of rash and, therefore, piperacillin-tazobactam should be avoided. This makes option B incorrect. Cefepime is a reasonable antibiotic to recommend for empiric antibiotic therapy for febrile neutropenia and JP does not have

any specific factors that would preclude use. Cefepime is a fourth-generation cephalosporin with a dissimilar R-1 side chain compared to penicillin making the potential cross reactivity very low. Thus, option C is correct. This patient also has a past medical history of epilepsy and is currently on divalproex sodium. A drug–drug interaction exists between divalproex sodium (i.e. valproic acid) and meropenem since carbapenem antibiotics can decrease valproic acid serum concentrations resulting in a lower seizure threshold and increasing the risk of seizures. Therefore, meropenem should be avoided in this case making answer choice D incorrect.

6. **Explanation:** The correct answer is B. Vancomycin is not routinely recommended as part of the initial empiric antibiotic regimen (i.e. in combination with an anti-pseudomonal beta-lactam).[1,2] Vancomycin (or another antibiotic targeted against gram-positive bacteria) is recommended in the following scenarios:

- Hemodynamic instability
- Positive blood cultures for gram-positive bacteria while awaiting speciation and susceptibility results
- Skin or soft tissue infection
- Pneumonia
- Suspected central venous catheter-related infection
- Severe mucositis if a patient was receiving fluoroquinolone prophylaxis lacking activity against streptococci and in those who are receiving ceftazidime as empiric therapy
- MRSA colonization or prior history of MRSA infection

While JP has a port in place, there was no erythema or tenderness noted on physical exam around the port site. It is important to remember that common signs and symptoms of infection may commonly be absent due to the blunted inflammatory response in neutropenic patients. Additionally, JP's MRSA nasal PCR results were negative.

7. **Explanation:** The correct answer is A. This demonstrates a catheter-related bloodstream infection, which is common in febrile neutropenia patients due to the presence of indwelling catheters for chemotherapy administration.[1,2] Blood cultures from peripheral sites and from the port are both growing *Pseudomonas aeruginosa*, which is susceptible to all of the antibiotics reported except ciprofloxacin. Catheter (ie, port) removal is recommended rather than salvaging the catheter for patients with catheter-related bloodstream infections caused by *Staphylococcus aureus*, *P. aeruginosa*, fungi, or mycobacteria. Therefore, the catheter/port should be removed making option C incorrect since salvaging the port and using antibiotic lock therapy are not recommended with *P. aeruginosa* catheter-related bloodstream infections. Option B is incorrect since we have susceptibility data and there is no need to broaden therapy to meropenem to cover for extended-spectrum beta-lactamase (ESBL)–producing bacteria as well as the drug–drug interaction with divalproex sodium. Option D is incorrect since we

TABLE 14.1.   Anti-Pseudomonal Beta-Lactam Dosing for Febrile Neutropenia in Patients with Normal Renal Function

Beta-Lactam	Dosing Regimen
Piperacillin-tazobactam	4.5 g IV every 6 hours
	3.375 g IV every 8 hours extended infusion
Cefepime	2 g IV every 8 hours
Ceftazidime	2 g IV every 8 hours
Meropenem	1 g IV every 8 hours
Imipenem-cilastatin	500 mg IV every 6 hours

have susceptibility data that reports cefepime as susceptible, so there is no need to add gentamicin and put the patient at an increased risk of nephrotoxicity. Therefore, option A is the correct answer since cefepime is susceptible and the catheter/port should be removed. The duration of therapy for uncomplicated catheter-related infections as described in this case is typically 14 days; however, data suggest that shorter courses of antibiotics may be sufficient.[3]

8. **Explanation:** The correct answer is A. In most cases, alterations to the initial empiric antibiotic regimen should be guided by clinical and microbiologic data.[1,2] However, empiric antifungal therapy and evaluation for invasive fungal infections should be considered in high-risk patients with persistent fevers after 4 to 7 days of appropriate antibiotics and when the duration of neutropenia is expected to be >7 days. An alternative antifungal agent

should be considered in patients who are currently receiving an antifungal agent for prophylaxis.

REFERENCES

1. Frefield AG, Bow EJ, Sepkowitz KA, et al. Clinical practice guideline for the use of antimicrobial agents in neutropenic patients with cancer: 2010 update by the Infectious Diseases Society of America. *Clin Infect Dis.* 2011;52:e56-e93.
2. Baden LR, Swaminathan S, Angarone M, et al. Prevention and treatment of cancer-related infections, version 2.2016, NCCN Clinical Practice Guidelines in Oncology. *J Natl Compr Canc Netw.* 2016;14(7):882-913.
3. Fabre V, Amoah J, Cosgrove SE, Tamma PD. Antibiotic therapy for *Pseudomonas aeruginosa* bloodstream infections: how long is long enough? *Clin Infect Dis.* 2019; 30882137. Epub ahead of print.

15 Skin and Soft Tissue Infection I

Michael Kelsch

PATIENT PRESENTATION

Chief Complaint

"My hand hurts really bad; it feels hot, like it is on fire."

History of Present Illness

SL is 25-year-old man who presents to the emergency department with worsening pain, redness, and swelling in his right hand. He got a splinter of wood on the palmer surface of his right hand near the base of his thumb 3 days ago while chopping wood. He thought he successfully removed the splinter, but the hand progressively became more painful and swollen where the splinter had been. Today, the burning pain (rated 8/10) has spread through his forearm and he is now feeling the pain up to his armpit. He reports that chills started yesterday. No numbness or tingling of the arm or hand, no weakness noted. Denies any prior issues with the hand.

Past Medical History

Recurrent major depressive disorder; ulnar neuropathy of left upper extremity secondary to motor vehicle accident 2 years ago; hepatitis C

Surgical History

Repair of anterior cruciate ligament in left knee in 2015; cholecystectomy in 2013; motor vehicle accident 2 years ago resulted in anterior cervical disc fusion C6/7, and repair of cervical fractures

Family History

Father has COPD; mother is healthy

Social History

Single; lives with friends; mechanic work occasionally in the past, but is currently unemployed. Smokes 1 ppd × 7 years and drinks 1 case of beer per week. Smokes marijuana, and inhales or injects methamphetamine daily.

Allergies

Penicillin (rash); sulfa (hives); morphine (itching)

Home Medications

Duloxetine 60 mg PO daily (nonadherent)
Amitriptyline 50 mg PO at bedtime (nonadherent)
Albuterol metered-dose-inhaler 1 to 2 puffs q4h PRN shortness of breath (nonadherent)

Physical Examination

> ### Vital Signs

Temp 98.8°F, HR 80 beats per minute, RR 16 breaths per minute, BP 127/83 mm Hg, pO_2 97% on room air; Ht 6'2″, Wt 67 kg

> ### General

He appears thin and not well nourished. Not significantly distressed, but somewhat anxious.

> ### HEENT

Normocephalic and atraumatic; no scleral icterus; normal range of motion; neck supple

> ### Pulmonary

Breath sounds normal. He has no wheezes or rales.

> ### Cardiovascular

Normal rate and regular rhythm; no murmur heard

> ### Abdomen

Soft; no tenderness

> ### Neurology

Alert and oriented to person, place, and time

> ### Skin

Skin is warm and dry, with scarring on various areas of extremities

> ### Musculoskeletal

Entry wound on the palmar surface near the base of the right thumb, scabbed over with surrounding erythema and swelling. No open wound or discharge. Swelling present throughout the right hand, including the dorsal surface. Hand very tender to palpation throughout. Brisk capillary refill. Pain with active and passive movement of hand. Extension and flexion of fingers mildly impaired due to swelling. Pain to palpation along forearm. Mild red streaking of the skin extending to the shoulder from the hand.

Laboratory Findings

Na = 136 mEq/L	Hgb = 13.9 g/dL	Ca = 8.8 mg/dL
K = 3.9 mEq/L	Hct = 42.6%	Mg = 1.9 mg/dL
Cl = 101 mEq/L	Plt = 226,000/mm³	Phos = 3.1 mg/dL
CO_2 = 29 mEq/L	WBC = 13,500/mm³	AST = 20 IU/L
BUN = 9 mg/dL	MCV = 98.2 fl/red cell	ALT = 39 IU/L
Cr = 0.83 mg/dL	ESR = 10 mm/hr	T Bili = 0.4 mg/dL
Glu = 90 mg/dL	CRP = 14.5 mg/L	Alk Phos = 86 IU/L
	CK = 93 U/L	Alb = 4 g/dL

► Urine Drug Screen

Positive for amphetamines, methamphetamine, benzodiazepines, marijuana, opiates, oxycodone

► Microbiology

Blood cultures × 2 (pending)
Culture (aerobic and anaerobic) of fluid from abscess on right hand (pending)

Imaging

MRI of right hand and lower right arm: (1) Abscess contacting the skin surface volar aspect hand between the fourth and fifth digits at level of the metacarpophalangeal joint. (2) Insinuating abscess dorsal hand and wrist. Connection between these 2 abscesses cannot be confirmed but could be too small to visualize. Possible concern for tenosynovitis. (3) No findings of osteoarthritis or septic arthritis within the hand or wrist

QUESTIONS

1. Which of the following findings from the clinical presentation correctly identifies the general type and severity of this skin infection?
   A. Purulent, mild
   B. Non-purulent, moderate
   C. Purulent, moderate
   D. Non-purulent, severe

2. Which of the following risk factors does SL have for community-acquired methicillin-resistant *Staphylococcus aureus* (CA-MRSA)?
   A. Injection drug use
   B. Cervical disc fusion 2 years ago
   C. Hepatitis C
   D. Mechanic work history

3. Which of the following interventions is considered most essential to ensure optimal management of this type of infection?
   A. Incision and drainage of the abscess
   B. Dressing changes of the infected area
   C. Decolonization of nares with intranasal mupirocin, and skin with chlorhexidine washes
   D. Anaerobic bacterial culture

4. Which empiric antimicrobial therapy is most appropriate for SL?
   A. Vancomycin
   B. Trimethoprim/sulfamethoxazole
   C. Daptomycin
   D. Ceftriaxone

5. Regardless of which antibiotic you chose in question 4, the attending physician would like to start vancomycin, pharmacy to dose. Please choose the most appropriate starting dose, and goal monitoring level, for SL.
   A. 1350 mg IV q12h; trough level of 10 to 20 mcg/mL prior to the 2nd dose
   B. 1350 mg IV q24h; trough level of 10 to 20 mcg/mL prior to the 4th dose
   C. 2000 mg IV q24h; peak level of 30 to 40 mcg/mL after the 4th dose
   D. 1000 mg IV q8h; trough level of 10 to 20 mcg/mL prior to the 4th dose

6. After 24 hours, SL's blood cultures show no growth. However, an aerobic culture of fluid from abscess drained on the right hand indicates moderate WBC (10 to 25/LPF), no epithelial cells, moderate gram-positive cocci in clusters (6 to 30 per OIF). An anaerobic culture of fluid from the abscess showed no growth. Which of the following bacteria will most likely be identified from this sample?
   A. *Streptococcus pyogenes*
   B. *Staphylococcus aureus*
   C. *Bacteroides fragilis*
   D. *Enterococcus faecalis*

7. What is the appropriate duration of antimicrobial treatment for this purulent skin infection that underwent successful incision and drainage?
   A. No antibiotics are necessary
   B. 4 to 7 days
   C. 7 to 14 days
   D. 4 to 6 weeks

8. The following chart represents the institution's outpatient antibiogram in relation to *Staphylococcus aureus*. Which

percentage represents this institution's CA-MRSA prevalence during this sampling period?

Staphylococcus aureus; total isolates = 1116

Antibiotic	Susceptibility (%)
Benzylpenicillin	20
Oxacillin	75
Gentamicin	99
Ciprofloxacin	79
Levofloxacin	80
Clindamycin	80
Erythromycin	58
Linezolid	100
Rifampin	99
Tetracycline	95
Trimethoprim/ Sulfamethoxazole	97
Vancomycin	100

A. 25%
B. 75%
C. 20%
D. 100%

9. SL reports feeling much better, still has pain but is manageable with pain medication, has been afebrile for the past 72 hours, blood cultures remain negative, and his wound appears to be healing well after the incision/drainage, IV antibiotics, and dressing changes. The physician would like to discharge this patient with oral antibiotics to complete the treatment regimen. Sensitivity results are displayed below. Which of the following oral antimicrobials is recommended for SL to complete his treatment regimen?

Organism: Staphylococcus aureus

Antibiotic	Value	Susceptibility
Clindamycin	≤0.25	Resistant
Erythromycin	≥8	Resistant
Levofloxacin	≥8	Resistant
Linezolid	≤2	Sensitive
Oxacillin	≥4	Resistant
Penicillin	≥0.5	Resistant
Rifampin	≤0.5	Sensitive
Tetracycline	≤1	Sensitive
Trimethoprim/ Sulfamethoxazole	≤10	Sensitive
Vancomycin	≤0.5	Sensitive

A. Linezolid
B. Doxycycline
C. Clindamycin
D. Trimethoprim/Sulfamethoxazole

ANSWERS

1. **Explanation:** The correct answer is C. Purulent abscess is discovered during physical examination. Purulent skin infections are predominately caused by *Staphylococcus aureus,* whereas nonpurulent infections are most often caused by *Streptococci* sp.[1] Patient's temperature on admission is 98.8°F; WBC = 13,500, HR = 80, RR = 16; therefore, he exhibits a systemic sign of infection (WBC > 12,000), which qualifies for at least moderate disease. Other signs of systemic infection include temperature >100.4, HR >90, and RR >24; this patient does not meet any of these criteria. It is moderate and not severe because he has not failed previous incision and drainage and antibiotics.[1]

2. **Explanation:** The correct answer is A. Injection drug use is an identified risk factor for CA-MRSA, as are tattoos and piercings, homelessness, HIV infection, men who have sex with men, and individuals who are routinely in close contact with others (athletic teams, dormitory occupants, military personnel, prison inmates, and child care centers).[2] Although this patient had a hospital stay post motor vehicle accident, it was 2 years ago and no longer is considered a risk factor for HA-MRSA since it is past the 90-day timeframe for it to be considered a risk factor. Hepatitis C itself is not considered a risk factor for CA-MRSA, nor is his occasional work as a mechanic.[2]

3. **Explanation:** The correct answer is A. Incision and drainage is the recommended treatment for abscesses.[1] Although dressing changes may improve wound healing, they are not more important than incision and drainage and antimicrobial therapy for skin abscess recovery. Decolonization is not warranted in this case; this is not a recurrent infection.[2] Also, decolonization is not part of acute infection management.[1] Anaerobic bacterial cultures may be beneficial for pathogen identification; however, incision and drainage is essential for source eradication and control.

4. **Explanation:** The correct answer is A. The decision to administer antibiotics directed against *S. aureus* as an adjunct to incision and drainage should be made based upon presence or absence of systemic inflammatory response syndrome (SIRS), such as temperature >38°C or <36°C, tachypnea >24 breaths per minute, tachycardia >90 beats per minute, or white blood cell count >12,000 or <400 cells/μL.[1] An antibiotic active against MRSA is recommended for patients who have failed initial antibiotic treatment or have markedly impaired host defenses or in patients with SIRS and hypotension.[1] Vancomycin is most appropriate because of its coverage of gram-positive bacteria including MRSA, in addition to the rapid spread of the infection demonstrated by the

patient symptoms and markedly elevated WBC count. Trimethoprim/sulfamethoxazole is incorrect because, although it covers many isolates of MRSA, its reliability is generally lower than vancomycin and is not endorsed by the IDSA MRSA treatment guidelines for hospitalized patients with a complicated SSTI (eg, patients with deeper soft-tissue infections, surgical/ traumatic wound infection, major abscesses, cellulitis, and infected ulcers and burns).[2] Ceftriaxone does not cover MRSA and is primarily used empirically for moderate nonpurulent skin infections because of its excellent coverage of *Streptococci* sp.[1] Although daptomycin covers MRSA, its usage is typically reserved for patients with MRSA isolates resistant to vancomycin, or when vancomycin is not tolerated (type 1 hypersensitivity reactions).[1]

5. **Explanation:** The correct answer is D. Vancomycin 15 to 20 mg/kg/dose (actual body weight) given IV every 8 to 12 h, not to exceed 2 g/dose, is recommended in patients with normal renal function. Some experts suggest vancomycin loading doses (25 mg/kg) for serious suspected or documented MRSA infections (sepsis, meningitis, pneumonia, or endocarditis) to enable early achievement of target trough concentrations, although clinical data are lacking.[3] Trough vancomycin concentrations are the most practical method to guide vancomycin dosing, although an AUC/MIC of >400 has been promoted as the ideal target to predict successful organism eradication.[3] There is not currently a widely accepted method to operationalize AUC/MIC monitoring. Serum trough concentrations should be obtained at steady-state conditions, prior to the fourth dose. This patient has normal renal function which should allow for vancomycin to reach steady state around the fourth dose. Patients with impaired renal function may not necessarily reach steady-state concentrations after the fourth dose and will likely require more frequent monitoring. Monitoring of peak vancomycin concentrations is not recommended as they do not correlate with therapeutic outcomes or toxicity.[3] For serious infections, such as bacteremia, infective endocarditis, osteomyelitis, meningitis, pneumonia, and severe SSTI (eg, necrotizing fasciitis) due to MRSA, vancomycin trough concentrations of 15 to 20 mcg/mL is recommended; otherwise trough concentrations of 10 to 15 mcg/mL are acceptable for nonserious infections.[1,3] SL's creatinine clearance is estimated at 129 mL/min using the original Cockcroft–Gault equation. SL's creatinine clearance and age warrant the empiric every 8-hour interval.

6. **Explanation:** The correct answer is B. Gram-positive cocci in clusters represent *Staphylococcus aureus,* which is the predominant bacteria involved in purulent skin infections. *Streptococcus pyogenes,* a gram-positive bacteria that is found in chains, is the predominant bacteria involved in nonpurulent skin infections.[1] *Enterococcus faecalis* is a gram-positive bacteria that is often found in short chains or diplococci and is not commonly found in skin infections. *Bacteroides fragilis* is a gram-positive, rod-shaped, anaerobic bacteria which most commonly is found in intra-abdominal infections, particularly those with abscess formation. Cutaneous abscesses may be polymicrobial, containing regional skin flora or organisms from the adjacent mucous membranes, but *S. aureus* alone causes a large percentage of skin abscesses, with a substantial number due to MRSA strains.[1,2]

7. **Explanation:** The correct answer is C. The duration of therapy for skin infections has not been well-defined, although no differences in outcome were observed among adult patients with uncomplicated cellulitis receiving 5 versus 10 days of therapy in a randomized, controlled trial. In the FDA licensing trials for complicated skin infections (as in this case), patients were typically treated for 7 to 14 days.[1] Duration of therapy should be individualized on the basis of the patient's clinical response. Four to 6 weeks is not warranted since this patient does not exhibit septic arthritis or osteomyelitis on MRI. Four to 7 days is an insufficient treatment duration, since the patient is not exclusively managed as an outpatient, does exhibit signs/symptoms of extensive disease (tenosynovitis concern on MRI), had rapid disease progression, has a history of injectable drug abuse (comorbid condition), and the abscess is on the hand area which may be difficult to completely drain.[1] No antibiotics is incorrect because of the extensive factors listed above. Incision and drainage alone may be warranted in mild outpatient cases where no signs and symptoms of systemic infection are present.[1]

8. **Explanation:** The correct answer is A. *Staphylococcus aureus* isolates are uncommonly susceptible to penicillin. Penicillin resistance (MSSA) is conferred by penicillinase production, which can be overcome by the addition of a beta-lactamase inhibitor (eg, amoxicillin/clavulanate, ampicillin/sulbactam) or use of penicillinase-resistant penicillin (eg, oxacillin, nafcillin).[1] Methicillin resistance is conferred by the presence of the *mecA* gene that encodes penicillin-binding protein 2a, an enzyme that has low affinity for beta-lactams and thus leads to resistance to methicillin, oxacillin, nafcillin, and cephalosporins in general except for ceftaroline.[2] Resistance percentage is calculated by taking 100% minus the susceptibility percentage of the particular antibiotic, in this case 100% − 75% (oxacillin) = 25%. Oxacillin is commonly used by laboratories to represent methicillin.

9. **Explanation:** The correct answer is B. Doxycycline is the most correct answer in this case considering that this MRSA isolate is susceptible. The isolate is resistant to clindamycin. Trimethoprim/sulfamethoxazole would be an option in this case based upon susceptibility results; however, this patient has an allergy to this antibiotic (rash). Linezolid would also be an option based upon susceptibility results; however, this patient abuses methamphetamine which increases neurotransmitters such as norepinephrine, dopamine, and serotonin. Linezolid is a weak monoamine oxidase inhibitor and therefore an

interaction may exist which potentially could generate dangerous levels of neurotransmitters and potentially cause sequela such as serotonin syndrome and hypertensive urgency/emergency.[4] Additionally, linezolid is more costly than doxycycline and trimethoprim/sulfamethoxazole and should be reserved for infections that do not respond to first-line therapy.[1,2]

REFERENCES

1. Stevens DL, Bisno AL, Chambers HF, et al. Guidelines for the Diagnosis and Management of Skin and Soft Tissue Infections: 2014 Update by the Infectious Diseases Society of America. *Clin Infect Dis.* 2014;59(2):e10-e52.

2. Liu C, Bayer A, Cosgrove SE, et al. Clinical Practice Guidelines by the Infectious Diseases Society of America for the Treatment of Methicillin-Resistant Staphylococcus aureus Infections in Adults and Children. *Clin Infect Dis.* 2011;52(3):e18-e55.

3. Rybak M, Lomaestro B, Rotschafer JC, et al. Therapeutic monitoring of vancomycin in adult patients: A consensus review of the American Society of Health-System Pharmacists, the Infectious Diseases Society of America, and the Society of Infectious Diseases Pharmacists. *Am J Health-Syst Pharm.* 2009;66:82-98.

4. Quinn DK, Stern TA. Linezolid and Serotonin Syndrome. *Prim Care Companion J Clin Psychiatry.* 2009;11(6):353-356.

16 Skin and Soft Tissue Infection II

Madeline King

PATIENT PRESENTATION

Chief Complaint

"I fell while hiking this weekend and now my arm has really a painful blister."

History of Present Illness

SP is a 36-year-old woman who presents to the emergency room of her local hospital 3 days after falling during a hike and sustaining an injury to her right upper extremity. She has a few scratches on her right lower extremity, but no punctures to the skin, scabs, or blisters. She has been taking acetaminophen 500 mg a few times per day since the fall, but states that it hasn't helped much. She also states that she washed the wound when she got home with soap and water, but didn't use hydrogen peroxide or apply any topical antibiotics.

Past Medical History

Seasonal allergies

Surgical History

None

Family History

Mother with hypertension
Father with diabetes
Maternal grandfather with heart failure

Social History

No illicit drug use
No tobacco use
Occasional alcohol use (2 to 3 times per month)

Allergies

NKDA

Home Medications

Ethinyl estradiol and norgestimate (Sprintec), 1 tablet by mouth daily
Fexofenadine (Allegra) 180 mg by mouth daily for allergies
Fluticasone (Flonase) nasal spray, one spray in each nostril twice daily during allergy season

Vitals on Admission

Temp 39.5°C, BP 111/54 mm Hg, P 86, RR 16 breaths per minute, Wt 57.5 kg, Ht 5'5"

Physical Examination

> #### General

Well-developed, well-nourished appearing Caucasian woman in no acute distress

> #### Skin

Right upper arm: red, erythematous, warm, and tender to touch; localized fluid collection that appears fluctuant

> #### HEENT

PERRLA; EOMI, oropharynx clear

> #### Neck/Lymph Nodes

Supple, no lymphadenopathy

> #### Lungs/Thorax

Clear to auscultation, no rales or wheezing

> #### Cardiovascular

Regular rate/rhythm, no murmurs/rubs/gallops

> #### Abdomen

Soft, NT/ND; (+) Bowel sounds

> #### Genitourinary/Rectal

No observed abnormalities

> #### Musculoskeletal/Extremities

Upper extremities: erythematous area on RUE with 2 × 3 cm abscess that is painful to touch
Lower extremities: no observed abnormalities

> #### Neurologic

A & O ×3

Imaging

X-ray of RUE: diffuse soft tissue swelling of upper arm; no subcutaneous gas or foreign body; no fractures

Laboratory Findings

WBC 18.1 × 10³ cells/μL	Plt 250,000/μL	Na 135 mEq/L
K 4.8 mEq/L	Glu 80 mg/dL	BUN 15
SCr 0.8 mg/dL		

QUESTIONS

1. Which structural component of the skin is MOST likely to be affected by cellulitis?
   A. Dermis
   B. Stratum corneum
   C. Fascia
   D. Bone

2. What organism is MOST commonly the cause of *purulent* skin/soft tissue infections?
   A. *Streptococcus pyogenes*
   B. *Staphylococcus aureus*
   C. *Pseudomonas aeruginosa*
   D. *Peptostreptococcus* spp.

3. How would you classify the severity of SP's infection?
   A. Mild
   B. Moderate
   C. Severe
   D. Life threatening

4. What would be the MOST appropriate empiric therapy for a patient with moderate purulent cellulitis?
   A. Incision and drainage plus doxycycline
   B. Incision and drainage plus dicloxacillin
   C. Amoxicillin
   D. Vancomycin

5. What definitive antibiotic therapy would be most appropriate for SP, assuming she does not need to be admitted to the hospital and cultures from the I&D result as methicillin susceptible *S. aureus*?
   A. Doxycycline
   B. Vancomycin
   C. Amoxicillin
   D. Dicloxacillin

6. What is the most appropriate treatment duration for SP?
   A. 5 days
   B. 10 days
   C. 14 days
   D. 21 days

7. Regardless of the antibiotic chosen in question 5, which adverse reactions would you need to counsel SP on if doxycycline was prescribed?
   A. *C. difficile* infection, Stevens–Johnson syndrome, anaphylaxis
   B. Photosensitivity, esophagitis
   C. Worsening infection, bone marrow suppression, GI upset
   D. Bone marrow suppression, acute kidney injury

ANSWERS

1. **Explanation:** The correct answer is A. Cellulitis can occur at any anatomical site and is characterized by redness and pain or swelling, except in the case of purulent cellulitis, which can also include abscesses and blisters. This is often the result of minor trauma, an abrasion, or after surgery. Cellulitis typically affects the dermis, while erysipelas affects the epidermis (rules out answer choice B). If the fascia is affected, that would be a more severe condition affecting deeper structural layers and leading to necrosis (eg, necrotizing fasciitis), thus ruling out answer choice C. Bone involvement would be the result of trauma going through multiple structural layers or a progressive, untreated SSTI which reached the bone, thus ruling out answer choice D.

2. **Explanation:** The correct answer is B. *S. pyogenes* is a common cause of nonpurulent cellulitis, including necrotizing fasciitis, and can produce toxins, thus ruling out answer choice A. *P. aeruginosa* is an uncommon cause of SSTI, except in some diabetic foot infections if the patient soaks his or her feet in water (as *P. aeruginosa* is commonly found in water sources), thus ruling out answer choice C. *Peptostreptococcus* is an anaerobic gram-positive coccus, which is normal flora of the mouth and genitourinary tract, and is more commonly seen in mixed infections, causing dental abscesses or genitourinary abscesses. It can cause cellulitis or other soft tissue infections, but these are less common, ruling out answer choice D. *S. aureus* is a common cause of purulent cellulitis.[1]

3. **Explanation:** The correct answer is B. Moderate severity: Purulent infection with signs of systemic inflammation (elevated WBC, fever, elevated HR, low BP). Other signs of systemic infection would include temperature >100.4°F and RR >24 breaths per minute. Since there are systemic signs of infection, this is not a mild infection, ruling out answer choice A. It is not severe because he has not failed previous therapy with incision and drainage (I&D) plus antibiotics, nor does he have progressive signs of a systemic response (eg, worsening temperature, blood pressure, heart rate, WBC), thus ruling out answer choices C and D.[1] It is important to determine severity because that will guide therapy choices. Mild infection requires only I&D, whereas moderate and severe infections require I&D with antibiotics given either orally or intravenously.

4. **Explanation:** The correct answer is A. Assume *S. aureus,* and the potential for methicillin-resistant *S. aureus* (MRSA) even in the community setting due to an increasing prevalence. Empiric treatment may be broad but should be narrowed once culture results are available.

Because we have to consider MRSA as a potential pathogen, we need an MRSA active agent empirically.[2] Doxycycline and vancomycin are the only two choices that cover MRSA, ruling out answer choices B and C.[1,2] For purulent cellulitis (or any infection with an abscess or other drainable/removable source, the first step is source control). Therefore, vancomycin without I&D is not the correct answer, but would be acceptable if a patient required intravenous (IV) antibiotics in addition to I&D (rules out answer choice D). Vancomycin should be dosed as 15 mg/kg every 12 hours, with a goal trough of 10 to 15 mcg/mL. I&D plus dicloxacillin would be correct if the pathogen is known to be methicillin-susceptible *S. aureus* (MSSA). Amoxicillin rarely covers *S. aureus* (most isolates are resistant to penicillin, ampicillin, amoxicillin due to production of a penicillinase). Additionally, even if it were susceptible, the patient would first require I&D. Therefore, doxycycline 100 mg twice daily would be the best choice.[1] An alternative option, not listed here, would be trimethoprim-sulfamethoxazole (TMP-SMX).

5. **Explanation:** The correct answer is D. Because you know now that the patient has MSSA, she doesn't need MRSA coverage any longer. It is most appropriate to use a narrower spectrum agent when possible. Of the listed options, vancomycin and doxycycline cover MRSA, which is not necessary, so A and B are not correct. As discussed in question 4, amoxicillin rarely covers *S. aureus,* ruling out option C. Susceptibilities were not provided, but most reports do not include penicillin or amoxicillin as options because of the rarity of susceptibility. Therefore, dicloxacillin, as an oral MSSA active agent, is the best option, dosed at 500 mg 4 times daily. Oral cephalosporins (eg, cephalexin) would also be viable options for MSSA. Doxycycline or trimethoprim-sulfamethoxazole would be appropriate oral options, despite having broader (eg, MRSA) coverage, and may be useful for patients with a penicillin allergy.[1]

6. **Explanation:** The correct answer is C. The recommended duration of antibiotic therapy for moderate, purulent cellulitis is 5 days unless there is a delay in clinical improvement, in which case the treatment duration could be extended. Clinical assessment should be used to determine why the patient is not improving and explore other reasons for continued disease. The benefits of shorter durations of therapy include a lower risk of adverse effects from antibiotics (eg, *Clostridioides difficile* infection), and preventing the emergence of resistance by providing unnecessary antibiotics.[3–6] If this were a mild infection, no antibiotics would be required.

7. **Explanation:** The correct answer is B. Any antibiotic could potentially cause *C. difficile* infection; however, certain antibiotics and longer courses of antibiotics cause an increased risk. Clindamycin has the highest risk of causing *C. difficile,* followed by cephalosporins and fluoroquinolones.[6] Although patients could develop an allergic reaction or anaphylaxis to any agent, allergies are more commonly reported for beta-lactams and TMP-SMX (answer choice A). TMP-SMX or linezolid would be the most likely antibiotics to cause bone marrow suppression (answer choices C and D). TMP-SMX is also one of the most likely to cause Stevens–Johnson syndrome (answer choice A).[7] Doxycycline can cause drug-induced esophagitis and photosensitivity; patients should be counseled to take doxycycline with a full glass of water, remain upright for at least 30 minutes after administration, and avoid prolonged sun exposure.[8] Therefore, the correct answer is B, photosensitivity, nausea, and esophagitis.

REFERENCES

1. Stevens DL, et al. Practice guidelines for the diagnosis and management of skin and soft tissue infections: 2014 update by the Infectious Diseases Society of America. *Clin Infect Dis.* 2014:59.
2. Horseman M, Bowman JD. Is community-acquired methicillin-resistant *Staphylococcus aureus* coverage needed for cellulitis? *Infect Dis Ther.* 2013;2:175-185.
3. Hepburn MJ, Dooley DP, Skidmore PJ, Ellis MW, Starnes WF, Hasewinkle WC. Comparison of short-course (5 days) and standard (10 days) treatment for uncomplicated cellulitis. *Arch Intern Med.* 2004;164(15):1669-1674.
4. Prokocimer P, De Anda C, Fang E, Mehra P, Das A. Tedizolid phosphate vs linezolid for treatment of acute bacterial skin and skin structure infections: the ESTABLISH-1 randomized trial. *JAMA.* 2013;309(6):559-569.
5. Moran GJ, Fang E, Corey GR, Das AF, De Anda C, Prokocimer P. Tedizolid for 6 days versus linezolid for 10 days for acute bacterial skin and skin-structure infections (ESTABLISH-2): a randomised, double-blind, phase 3, non-inferiority trial. *Lancet Infect Dis.* 2014;14(8):696-705.
6. Brown KA. Meta-analysis of antibiotics and the risk of community-associated *Clostridium difficile* infection. *Antimicrob Agents Chemoth.* 2013;57(5):2326-2332.
7. Sulfamethoxazole-trimethoprim [package insert]. Kenner, LA: New Horizon Rx Group, LLC; 2013
8. Doxycycline [package insert]. Morgantown, WV: Mylan; 2019.

17 Necrotizing Fasciitis

Tianrui Yang   Jonathan C. Cho

PATIENT PRESENTATION

Chief Complaint

"My right leg hurts."

History of Present Illness

WL is a 52-year-old Caucasian male who presents to the emergency department with pain and redness of his lower right leg as well as fever and malaise. He also noticed bulla formation on his right shin which worsened within hours. He recalls accidentally bumping his leg on the side of his bed and sustaining an abrasion to his shin 2 days ago. He states he had to skip work the next day since it was so painful. When the pain got worse overnight, he decided to come into the emergency department.

Past Medical History

HTN, type 2 DM, HLD

Surgical History

Appendectomy

Family History

Father had CAD and passed away from a myocardial infarction at age 50; mother has type 2 DM and hypothyroidism.

Social History

Married and living with his wife. Smokes ½ ppd × 30 years and drinks alcohol socially.

Allergies

NKDA

Home Medications

Lisinopril 40 mg PO daily
Atorvastatin 80 mg PO daily
Metformin 1 g PO BID
Empagliflozin 25 mg PO daily

Physical Examination

▶ Vital Signs

Temp 102.4°F, P 107, RR 24 breaths per minute, BP 124/70 mm Hg, pO_2 97 %, Ht 5'11", Wt 100 kg

▶ General

Well-developed, well-nourished male; appears lethargic and in distress

▶ HEENT

Normocephalic, atraumatic, PERRLA, EOMI, normal funduscopic exam, normal visual fields

▶ Pulmonary

Clear to auscultation bilaterally, no rales/rhonchi/wheezes

▶ Cardiovascular

NSR, no m/r/g

▶ Abdomen

Soft, non-distended, non-tender, normal bowel sounds

▶ Genitourinary

Deferred; no complaints of dysuria or hematuria

▶ Neurology

Lethargic, oriented to place, person, and time

▶ Extremities

5 × 12 cm erythematous patch with bullae on the front RLE, tender to palpation

Laboratory Findings

Na 140 mEq/L	Ca 8.2 mg/dL	WBC 16.3 g/dL
K 3.7 mEq/L	Mg 2.1 mg/dL	Hgb 12.7 g/dL
Cl 103 mEq/L	PO_4 4.1 mg/dL	Hct 38%
HCO_3 26 mEq/L	AST 22 U/L	Plt 256 × 10^3/μL
BUN 19 mg/dL	ALT 15 U/L	
SCr 1.2 mg/dL	T Bili 0.9 mg/dL	
Glu 173 mg/dL	Alk Phos 81 U/L	
A1c 7.5%	Lactate 0.8 mmol/L	

▶ CT of RLE

Extensive gas formation in the soft tissues of the front leg along the fascial planes toward the back of the leg and the knee

▶ **Blood Cultures**

Pending

QUESTIONS

1. Which of the following is NOT a risk factor that WL has for contracting necrotizing fasciitis?
   A. Obesity
   B. Type 2 DM
   C. Injury
   D. HLD

2. Given WL's risk factors, which type(s) of necrotizing fasciitis is/are WL most at risk for contracting?
   A. Type I
   B. Type I & II
   C. Type II
   D. Type II & IV
   E. Type III

3. Which of the following is/are clinical features of necrotizing fasciitis?
   A. Tenderness only within the cutaneous erythema
   B. Presence of crepitus
   C. Rapid response to IV antibiotic therapy
   D. Mild pain without systemic signs or symptoms

4. How is necrotizing fasciitis best diagnosed?
   A. CT is the gold standard of diagnosis as it has great sensitivity and specificity for showing edema along the fascial plane
   B. MRI is the gold standard of diagnosis as it has great sensitivity and specificity for showing edema along the fascial plane
   C. Appearance of the subcutaneous tissues or fascial planes seen during surgical exploration
   D. Clinical scoring systems such as the laboratory risk indicator for necrotizing fasciitis (LRINEC)

5. What is an appropriate management plan for WL?
   A. Surgical debridement
   B. Surgical debridement along with antibiotics
   C. Surgical debridement along with antibiotics and aggressive fluid administration
   D. Surgical debridement along with antibiotics, aggressive fluid administration, and IVIG

6. Which of the following would be an appropriate initial antibiotic regimen?
   A. Piperacillin-tazobactam + vancomycin
   B. Meropenem
   C. Penicillin + clindamycin
   D. Ceftriaxone + linezolid

7. WL is stable after debridement and empiric antibiotics. His finalized tissue culture was only positive for group A *Streptococcus*. What is the most appropriate next course of action?
   A. Continue all antibiotics as diabetic patients are at risk for polymicrobial disease
   B. De-escalate to vancomycin alone

C. De-escalate to penicillin alone
D. De-escalate to penicillin + clindamycin

8. What is the appropriate duration of treatment for WL?
   A. 4 to 6 weeks of IV antibiotics
   B. A minimum of 2 weeks of IV antibiotics after last debridement
   C. A minimum of 2 weeks of IV antibiotics followed by 2 weeks of PO antibiotics
   D. Continued for a few days after patient is clinically improved, afebrile for at least 48 hours, and no longer needs debridement

9. Which of the following is NOT a potential complication that WL should be monitored for?
   A. Fournier gangrene
   B. Toxic shock syndrome
   C. Compartment syndrome
   D. Septic shock

ANSWERS

1. **Explanation:** The correct answer is D. Choices A through C are all identified risk factors for necrotizing fasciitis. Other risk factors to consider when screening patients include IV drug use, immunocompromised state, and chronic diseases such as renal failure, cirrhosis, and alcoholism.[1] Diabetes is recognized as a significant risk factor as 44.5% to 72.3% of necrotizing fasciitis patients have been reported to have diabetes as an underlying disease.[2] In most cases, clinical features of necrotizing fasciitis extend from a skin lesion. Injury ranges from large surgical incisions to small lesions such as insect bites or injection sites (ie, IVDU). However, a small percentage of the patients may have no visible skin lesion.[3]

2. **Explanation:** The correct answer is B. There are 4 types of necrotizing fasciitis.[4] Type I, or polymicrobial necrotizing fasciitis, is the most common type of the disease. Causative pathogens include a combination of gram-positive cocci, gram-negative rods, and anaerobes. Patients with Type I necrotizing fasciitis are typically older patients with comorbidities such as diabetes and peripheral vascular disease. Trauma may or may not be present in this type of necrotizing fasciitis. Type II infections involve group A β-hemolytic *Streptococcus*, with or without staphylococcal species. Type II infections tend to occur in younger patients. Risk factors for Type II infections include a history of trauma, surgery, or IVDU. Type III infections are caused by marine organisms, most commonly *Vibrio* spp. or *Clostridium* spp. *Vibrio* spp. are natural inhabitants of coastal waters in the southeastern United States, Central and South America, and Asia. *Clostridium* spp. are anaerobic bacteria that can result from intestinal surgical wounds or external wounds causing local devascularization. Type III infections typically occur through contamination of a pre-existing wound or through an injury acquired while exposed to salt water. However, ingestion of raw seafood has also been reported

to cause Type III infections. Type IV infections are caused by fungal organisms, typically *Candida* spp. Type IV infections are very rare and typically occur in patients with traumatic wounds and burns and in those who are severely immunocompromised. Given WL's PMH of DM and SH of IVDU, he is most at risk for developing Type I and Type II infections.

3. **Explanation:** The correct answer is B. Choice A is incorrect as patients with necrotizing fasciitis will typically experience edema or tenderness beyond the cutaneous erythema. Choice C is incorrect because patients with necrotizing fasciitis will typically fail to respond to initial antibiotic therapy (regardless of IV or PO) and develop progressive redness and swelling despite antibiotics (in contrast to cellulitis). Choice D is incorrect because these patients will typically experience severe pain that seems disproportional to the clinical findings. Other clinical features include hard, wooden feel of the subcutaneous tissue, bullous lesion, and skin necrosis or ecchymoses.[3]

4. **Explanation:** The correct answer is C. Although both CT and MRI may show edema extending along the fascial plane, the sensitivity and specificity of these studies are not well defined and may delay definitive diagnosis and treatment and therefore choices A and B are incorrect. Choice D is incorrect because while clinical scoring systems are useful aids for diagnosis, they should not be used as the gold standard for diagnosis as their accuracy in identifying necrotizing fasciitis produced conflicting results. In diagnosing necrotizing fasciitis, clinical features are important in raising the initial suspicion. To confirm the suspicion, the most important diagnostic feature is the appearance of the tissues seen during surgery. Findings include swollen and dull-gray appearance of the fascia, thin exudate without clear purulence, and easy separation of tissue planes by blunt dissection.[3]

5. **Explanation:** The correct answer is C. Treatment of necrotizing fasciitis will require surgical management. After initial debridement, patients should return to the operating room daily until the surgical team finds no further need for debridement. Antibiotics should also be administered in conjunction with surgical debridement to help treat and prevent the spread of infection. Since these wounds can discharge large amounts of tissue fluid, IV fluid replacement should be given to maintain adequate hydration.[3] Lastly, while IVIG may be beneficial in treating streptococcal infections by neutralizing the toxins, it should not be started empirically before the identification of the pathogen as data supporting use is inconsistent.[5]

6. **Explanation:** The correct answer is A. Treatment of necrotizing fasciitis should be based on the suspected type of infection. If Type I necrotizing fasciitis is suspected, broad-spectrum antibiotics effective against gram-positive organisms such as methicillin-resistant *S. aureus* (MRSA), gram-negative organisms such as *E. coli* and *Klebsiella* spp., and anaerobic organisms such as *Clostridium* and *Peptostreptococcus* spp. should be initiated. If Type II infection is suspected, a combination of penicillin and clindamycin is recommended. For Type III infections, a combination of third-generation cephalosporin and doxycycline or minocycline should be started. Lastly, antifungal therapy, such as fluconazole and amphotericin B, should be initiated if the patient has Type IV necrotizing fasciitis. The antifungal agent selected should be based on the suspected/isolated organism and susceptibility. Since fungal necrotizing fasciitis is rare and typically only occurs in patients who are severely immunocompromised, there is no need to add antifungal coverage for WL at this time. When there is not a clear suspicion for one type of infection, empiric therapy should be broad and provide coverage for gram-positive, gram-negative, and anaerobes.[3] MRSA coverage should be based on prevalence of MRSA in the region. Choice B is incorrect because meropenem lacks MRSA coverage. Choice C is incorrect because this regimen does not provide sufficient gram-negative coverage. Choice D is incorrect because this regimen does not cover anaerobic organisms.

7. **Explanation:** The correct answer is D. Choice A is incorrect because while diabetes is a risk factor for polymicrobial necrotizing fasciitis, this is not the case with WL as evidenced by the tissue culture, and antibiotics should be de-escalated for stewardship purposes. While vancomycin covers *Streptococcus* spp., choice B is incorrect since vancomycin is neither the narrowest option nor the treatment of choice for group A *Streptococcus* infections. Although penicillin is the treatment of choice for infections due to group A *Streptococcus*, choice C is not the best answer in this case since a combination therapy with clindamycin is recommended when treating necrotizing fasciitis caused by group A *Streptococcus*. Clindamycin is able to suppress toxin and cytokine production by group A *Streptococcus* through the inhibition of bacterial protein synthesis and potentially decrease skin necrosis.[3]

8. **Explanation:** The correct answer is D. There is no established time period for the duration of treatment. Duration is based on clinical status and the need for debridement as complete debridement is the only way to achieve source control.[3]

9. **Explanation:** The correct answer is A. Fournier gangrene is a variant of necrotizing soft tissue infection that involves the scrotum and penis or vulva. It's a similar disease but it's not considered a complication from the current disease that WL has (Fournier gangrene is typically caused by facultative organisms and anaerobes).[3] Toxic shock syndrome is an abrupt onset, life-threatening complication characterized by vascular collapse and multiorgan failure. WL is at risk for this because the causative pathogen for his necrotizing fasciitis is group A *Streptococcus* which can release toxins to cause toxic shock syndrome. Compartment syndrome is a painful condition that typically results from trauma. Necrotizing fasciitis

may cause tissue hypoxia, edema, and altered oxygen tension that lead to an increase in intracompartmental pressure resulting in tissue ischemia, necrosis, and nerve damage. Septic shock is another life-threatening complication characterized by vasodilatory hypotension despite fluid resuscitation and elevated lactate level and may arise from many different infections including necrotizing fasciitis.[6]

REFERENCES

1. Puvanendran R, Huey J, Pasupathy S. Necrotizing fasciitis. *Can Fam Physician*. 2009 Oct;55(10):981-987.
2. Cheng N, Tai H, Chang S, Chang C, Lai H. Necrotizing fasciitis in patients with diabetes mellitus: clinical characteristics and risk factors for mortality. *BMC Infect Dis*. 2015;15:417.
3. Stevens DL, Bisno AL, Chambers HF, et al. Practice guidelines for the diagnosis and management of skin and soft tissue infections: 2014 update by the Infectious Diseases Society of America. *Clin Infect Dis*. 2014;59(2):e10-e52.
4. Davoudian P, Flint N. Necrotizing fasciitis. *Anaesth Crit Care Pain*. 2012;12(5):245-250.
5. Parks T, Wilson C, Curtis N, Norrby-Teglund A, Sriskandan S. Polyspecific intravenous immunoglobulin in clindamycin-treated patients with streptococcal toxic shock syndrome: a systematic review and meta-analysis. *Clin Infect Dis*. 2018;67(9):1434.
6. Centers for Disease Control and Prevention. Necrotizing fasciitis: all you need to know. Available at https://www.cdc.gov/groupastrep/diseases-public/necrotizing-fasciitis.html. Atlanta, GA, 2018.

18 Diabetic Foot Infection

Kayla R. Stover

PATIENT PRESENTATION

Chief Complaint

"My foot is red, draining fluid, and it stinks."

History of Present Illness

EH is a 58-year-old female who presents to the hospital with a wound to the right plantar surface of the foot that is edematous, erythematous, and with foul-smelling drainage. She was seen in the emergency department 6 days ago and received clindamycin 300 mg every 8 hours for 5 days. She reports compliance with the medications, and has been soaking her feet routinely in hot water. Since that time, her wound has only worsened. She denies fever or chills but reports frequent feelings of hopelessness.

Past Medical History

Insulin-dependent type 2 diabetes, dyslipidemia, HTN, ESRD (on dialysis), depression, hypothyroidism, and CAD

Surgical History

AV fistula placement, cholecystectomy, coronary artery bypass graft, finger amputation, oophorectomy, tonsillectomy, and adenoidectomy

Family History

Father had diabetes, Alzheimer's disease, heart disease, HTN, high cholesterol, arthritis, and vision loss and passed away 2 years ago; mother has diabetes, HTN, high cholesterol, and history of stroke

Social History

Smokes ½ pack per day × 15 years; reports no alcohol or illicit drug use

Allergies

Penicillin (lip swelling, tongue irritation; has tolerated cephalosporins and carbapenems in the past); atorvastatin ("spaghetti legs"; tolerates pravastatin)

Home Medications

Allopurinol 100 mg PO daily
Amlodipine 10 mg PO daily
Aspirin 81 mg PO daily
B-complex-C-folic acid (RENA-VITE): 1 tablet PO daily
Calcitriol 0.25 mcg PO daily
Carvedilol 25 mg PO BID with meals
Cetirizine 10 mg PO daily
Furosemide 20 mg PO daily
Insulin glargine 35 units subcutaneously qHS
Insulin lispro 4 units subcutaneously TID before meals
Levothyroxine 50 mcg PO daily
Omeprazole 20 mg PO daily
Pravastatin 80 mg PO qHS
Sevelamer 3200 mg (4 tablets) PO TID with meals
Sertraline 100 mg PO daily

Physical Examination

> #### Vital Signs

Temp 98.3°F, P 66, RR 18 breaths per minute, BP 161/94 mm Hg, spO$_2$ 99%, Ht 5'4", Wt 81.1 kg

> #### General

Well-developed, well-nourished female oriented to person, place, and time

> #### HEENT

Normocephalic, atraumatic, external ears normal, oropharynx clear and moist; no discharge from eyes, no scleral icterus; neck supple

> #### Pulmonary

Effort and breath sounds normal; no respiratory distress

> #### Cardiovascular

RRR, normal heart sounds; no m/r/g

> #### Abdomen

Soft, bowel sounds normal

▶ *Musculoskeletal*

Right lower extremity reddened and edematous from ankle downward; +2 pedal pulses bilaterally

▶ *Skin*

Warm and dry. Foul smelling wound with yellow drainage noted to right plantar surface of foot. Macerated edges noted with surrounding redness and swelling.

▶ *Neurology*

Alert and oriented to person, place, and time

▶ *Psychiatric*

Normal mood and affect; behavior normal

Laboratory Findings

Na = 134 mEq/L   WBC = 6 × 10^3/mm³   ESR = 61.0 mm/hr

K = 5.0 mEq/L   Hgb = 10.3 g/dL   CRP = 2.30 mg/L

Cl = 90 mEq/L   Hct = 31.6%   PT 12.5 sec

CO_2 = 25 mEq/L   Plt = 206 × 10^3/mm³   INR 1.06

BUN = 57.0 mg/dL

Scr = 6.29 mg/dL

Glu = 246 mg/dL

▶ *X-ray Foot*

From ED visit: Medially prominent soft tissue swelling; erosive changes in the medial head of the first metatarsal, medial and lateral head of the second metatarsal, and lateral head of fifth metatarsal; erosive changes could be consistent with known neuropathic arthropathy.

▶ *Blood Cultures*

Pending

▶ *Deep Wound/Tissue Cultures*

Pending

QUESTIONS

1. Based on presentation, how would this patient be classified according to the systems developed by the International Working Group on the Diabetic Foot (PEDIS grade) and the Infectious Diseases Society of America?
   A. 1, uninfected
   B. 2, mild
   C. 3, moderate
   D. 4, severe

2. In addition to the evaluation of signs and symptoms on presentation, which of the following tests would be most helpful to diagnose a patient with a diabetic foot infection?
   A. C-reactive protein
   B. Erythrocyte sedimentation rate
   C. Magnetic resonance imaging
   D. White blood count

3. Which of the following types of pathogen would you suspect is responsible for EH's diabetic foot infection?
   A. Aerobic gram-negative bacilli
   B. Aerobic gram-positive cocci
   C. Anaerobic organisms
   D. All of the above

4. Which of the following best describes the risk factors for acquiring diabetic foot infections caused by *Pseudomonas aeruginosa*?
   A. Chronic, previously treated wounds now with severe infection
   B. High local prevalence, warm climate, frequent water exposure
   C. Nasal carriage, previous hospitalization, and local resistance
   D. Prior long-term antibiotic use and long duration of foot wound

5. Which specific factor is most likely to put EH at risk for a drug-resistant pathogen?
   A. Complicated past medical history
   B. History of smoking ½ pack per day
   C. Previous treatment with clindamycin
   D. Previous visit to the emergency department

6. Which of the following regimens would be the best empiric therapy for EH?
   A. Amoxicillin-clavulanate orally
   B. Ciprofloxacin plus metronidazole orally
   C. Clindamycin plus penicillin intravenously
   D. Vancomycin plus piperacillin-tazobactam intravenously

7. EH responds well to initial therapy, with improvements in the appearance of her foot. Three days into therapy, deep wound cultures grow methicillin-susceptible *Staphylococcus aureus*. Which agent would be best to recommend for EH?
   A. Daptomycin
   B. Dicloxacillin
   C. Levofloxacin
   D. Vancomycin

8. What would be the most appropriate duration of therapy for a severe diabetic foot infection with residual underlying bony involvement?
   A. 1 to 2 weeks
   B. 2 to 4 weeks
   C. 4 to 6 weeks
   D. ≥3 months

ANSWERS

1. **Explanation:** The correct answer is C. This patient meets the criteria for infection (erythema + edema + discharge; answer A is incorrect), but has surrounding edema >2 cm (per physical exam, reddened and swollen from ankle downward), placing them into Grade 3 or moderate infection (answer B is incorrect). This patient has no signs or symptoms of systemic infection, so would not be classified as severe (Grade 4) (answer D is incorrect).[1]

Diabetic Foot Infection Severity Classification by the IDSA and PEDIS Grading Scales		
IDSA Severity	**PEDIS Grade**	**Signs/Symptoms**
Uninfected	1	No signs or symptoms of infection[a]
Mild	2	Local infection (no involvement of deeper tissues); erythema between 0.5 and 2 cm
Moderate	3	Local infection with erythema >2 cm or involvement of deeper tissues/structures WITHOUT signs of systemic inflammatory response syndrome (SIRS)[b]
Severe	4	Local infection plus signs of SIRS[b]

IDSA, Infectious Diseases Society of America; PEDIS, International Working Group on the Diabetic Foot Infection.
[a]To be defined as an infection, 2 or more of the following should be present: local swelling or induration, erythema, local tenderness or pain, local warmth, purulent discharge.
[b]To be defined as SIRS, 2 or more of the following should be present: temperature >38°C or <36°C, heart rate >90 beats per minute, respiratory rate >20 breaths per minute or $PaCO_2$ <32 mm Hg, white blood count >12,000 or <4000 cells/μL or ≥10% immature forms.
Source: Data from Lipsky BA, Berendt AR, Cornia PB, et al.; Infectious Diseases Society of America. 2012 Infectious Diseases Society of America clinical practice guideline for the diagnosis and treatment of diabetic foot infections. *Clin Infect Dis.* 2012;54(12):e132-e73.

2. **Explanation:** The correct answer is C. Although C-reactive protein, erythrocyte sedimentation rate, and white blood counts are laboratory markers suggestive of infection, they are not specific to diabetic foot infection (answers A, B, and D are incorrect). In contrast, radiography including both plan films (X-ray) and magnetic resonance imaging (MRI) are recommended by the guidelines in order to identify bony abnormalities, soft tissue gas, foreign bodies, and/or deeper, underlying infections such as osteomyelitis.[1]

3. **Explanation:** The correct answer is D. Based on EH's medical and surgical history and reports of previous treatment that failed (6 days on clindamycin from the emergency department), she likely has frequent health care exposure, which puts her at higher risk for polymicrobial infection with gram-positive, gram-negative, and anaerobic organisms (answers A, B, and C are incorrect).[1]

4. **Explanation:** The correct answer is B. According to the IDSA clinical practice guidelines, warm climates, frequent exposure to water, and high local prevalence of *Pseudomonas aeruginosa* increase the risk of infection with that pathogen.[1] Chronic wounds or those that have been previously treated or that are with severe infection are most likely representative of anaerobic organisms (answer A is incorrect). Risk factors for methicillin-resistant *Staphylococcus aureus* (MRSA) include prior long-term or inappropriate use of antibiotics, previous hospitalizations, long duration of foot wounds, presence of osteomyelitis, and nasal carriage of MRSA (answers C and D are incorrect).

5. **Explanation:** The correct answer is C. Previous antibiotic use or treatment failure is a specific risk factor for infection with drug-resistant pathogens, including methicillin-resistant *Staphylococcus aureus.*[1] Although previous hospitalizations are also risk factors, this does not include outpatient visits (such as to the emergency department) (answer D is incorrect). Although a complicated past medical and smoking history are potentially risk factors for complications, they have not specifically been associated with drug resistance (answers A and B are incorrect).

6. **Explanation:** The correct answer is D. For moderate to severe infections, the guidelines suggest starting with intravenous therapy that is sufficiently broad to cover suspected pathogens.[1] This patient has potential risk factors for both methicillin-resistant *Staphylococcus aureus* and *Pseudomonas aeruginosa,* so should be covered for both empirically. For mild or some moderate infections, oral therapy would be appropriate. This patient has previously failed oral therapy, so she should be started initially on intravenous therapy (answers A and B are incorrect). In addition, amoxicillin-clavulanate is a suggested therapy only for mild infection. Although ciprofloxacin plus metronidazole would cover gram-negative and anaerobic pathogens, that regimen would not cover *Staphylococcus aureus,* which may be a factor for this patient. Clindamycin is an option for mild infections, but this patient already failed therapy. In addition, clindamycin plus penicillin would not cover the most suspected pathogens (answer C is incorrect).

7. **Explanation:** The correct answer is B. Dicloxacillin provides specific, targeted therapy toward methicillin-susceptible *Staphylococcus aureus* (MSSA). This patient has responded well to initial therapy (defined as improvement in or resolution of signs or symptoms of infection

[redness, swelling, induration, pain, purulence] and/or improvement or resolution of SIRS criteria [normalization of temperature, white blood count, heart rate, and respiratory rate]), and culture results are back, meeting the criteria for conversion to oral therapy according to the diabetic foot infection guidelines.[1] Daptomycin and vancomycin would both provide intravenous options, but are broader spectrum agents than are needed for MSSA (answers A and D are incorrect). Although levofloxacin provides a nice oral option, the guidelines suggest it is suboptimal against *Staphylococcus aureus* and an alternative should be selected (answer C is incorrect).

8. **Explanation:** The correct answer is C. The guidelines recommend 4 to 6 weeks of therapy for patients with diabetic foot infection with residual underlying bony involvement.[1] Mild to moderate infections may be treated for 1 to 3 weeks (answer A is incorrect), while severe infections without residual bony involvement may be treated for 2 to 4 weeks (answer B is incorrect). Only patients with severe infection with residual dead bone should be treated for 3 or more months (answer D is incorrect).

Route, Duration, and Treatment Location for Diabetic Foot Infections			
Classification	**Route**	**Duration**	**Treatment Location**
Mild	Topical or oral	1–2 weeks	Outpatient
Moderate	Oral or initial IV	1–3 weeks	Outpatient or Inpatient
Severe	Initial IV, switch to oral when possible	2–4 weeks	Inpatient then Outpatient
Bone involvement with amputation	IV or oral	2–5 days	Inpatient then Outpatient
Bone involvement with residual infected bone	Initial IV, switch to oral when possible	4–6 weeks	Inpatient then outpatient
Bone involvement with residual necrotic bone	Initial IV, switch to oral when possible	≥3 months	Inpatient then outpatient

Source: Data from Lipsky BA, Berendt AR, Cornia PB, et al; Infectious Diseases Society of America. 2012 Infectious Diseases Society of America clinical practice guideline for the diagnosis and treatment of diabetic foot infections. *Clin Infect Dis.* 2012;54(12):e132-e73.

REFERENCE

1. Lipsky BA, Berendt AR, Comia PB, et al. 2012 Infectious Diseases Society of America clinical practice guidelines for the diagnosis and treatment of diabetic foot infections. *Clin Infect Dis.* 2012;54:132-173.

19 Vertebral Osteomyelitis

Meghan N. Jeffres

PATIENT PRESENTATION

Chief Complaint

Back pain

History of Present Illness

CJ is a 62-year-old male who was referred to the hospital by his primary care physician for further workup for back pain. His back pain started six weeks ago and has gotten progressively worse over that time. Stretching and exercise have not helped with the pain. Lying flat in bed provides some relief. The pain is localized to his lower back and gets worse throughout the day. The pain was severe during his physical exam this morning, which is why he was referred to the hospital for further workup. He denies nausea, vomiting, fevers, chills, chest pain, shortness of breath, and bowel or bladder incontinence.

Past Medical History

Hyperlipidemia, hypertension

Family History

Noncontributory

Social History

Denies illicit substances; consumes EtOH socially—approximately three 12 oz beers weekly; lives with his wife of 35 years; employed as an electrician

Allergies

NKDA

Home Medications

Atorvastatin 40 mg PO daily
Lisinopril 40 mg PO daily
Acetaminophen 500 mg PO PRN for back pain
Ibuprofen 400 mg PO PRN for back pain; he has increased use of APAP and ibuprofen over the past 6 weeks

Physical Examination

▶ **Vital Signs**

Temp 98.4°F, BP 151/98 mm Hg, P 83 bpm, RR 14 breaths per minute, 96% O_2 situation on room air, Ht 5′9″, Wt 90 kg

▶ **General**

He does not appear to be in any acute distress

▶ **HEENT**

Pupils equal/round, reactive to light, conjunctiva clear; poor dentition noted

▶ **Pulmonary**

Clear to auscultation bilaterally, no wheezing, rhonchi, or rales

▶ **Cardiovascular**

Regular rate and rhythm; no appreciable murmurs, gallops, or rubs

▶ **Abdominal**

Soft, non-tender, non-distended; bowel sounds present

▶ **Genital/Rectal**

Exam deferred

▶ **Extremities**

No edema; peripheral pulses intact; normal range of motion; no evidence of injection sites or skin infection

▶ **Back**

He has reproducible pain in the lumbar spine.

▶ **Neurologic**

Cranial nerves II–XII are intact. Alert and oriented × 3; mood, affect appropriate

Laboratory Findings

Na 131 mEq/L	Hgb 14.1 g/dL	AST 35 IU/L
K 4.2 mEq/L	Hct 42%	ALT 40 IU/L
Cl 97 mEq/L	Plt 498 × 10^3/mm³	Alk Phos 80 IU/L
CO_2 24 mEq/L	WBC 12.3 × 10^3/mm³	T Bili 1.4 mg/dL
BUN 19 mg/dL	Neutros 77%	
SCr 1.1 mg/dL	Bands 17%	ESR 103 mm/hr
Glucose 89 mg/dL	Lymphs 4%	CRP 76 mg/L
Ca 9.4 mg/dL	Monos 8%	
Mg 2.1 mg/dL		

▶ **CT Scan**

CT scan of abdomen and pelvis are unremarkable. Lumbar spine shows degenerative disc disease.

▶ **MRI**

T1-weighted–decreased signal intensity in lumbar vertebral bodies and disc; T2-weighted–increased disc signal intensity. Impression: osteomyelitis of lumbar spine, no evidence of abscess

▶ **Blood and Urine Cultures**

Pending

QUESTIONS

1. What is the most likely source of CJ's vertebral osteomyelitis?
   A. Skin infection
   B. IV drug use
   C. Poor dentition
   D. Diverticulitis flare

2. What is CJ's primary symptom of vertebral osteomyelitis?
   A. Fever
   B. Back pain
   C. Elevated ESR and CRP
   D. Hemodynamic instability

3. A physician in the emergency room saw CJ's MRI results and initiated vancomycin and piperacillin/tazobactam. While in the ED, CJ received 1 dose each of vancomycin and piperacillin/tazobactam before a biopsy of the infected bone was performed. How will the receipt of antibiotics affect the likelihood of growing a pathogen from the biopsy?
   A. Reduces microbiology yield by 25%
   B. Reduces microbiology yield by 50%
   C. Reduces microbiology yield by 90%
   D. No reduction in microbiology yield if biopsy is within 3 days of antibiotic receipt

4. When should empiric antibiotics be initiated for CJ?
   A. As soon as osteomyelitis is seen or suspected in imaging (CT, MRI, X-ray)
   B. After blood cultures obtained
   C. After bone biopsy is performed
   D. After bone biopsy, culture, and susceptibilities are complete

5. What pathogen(s) is/are the most common cause of vertebral osteomyelitis and should be covered in the setting of negative biopsy cultures or if biopsy is not performed?
   A. Streptococci
   B. *Staphylococcus aureus*
   C. Gram-negative bacilli
   D. *Mycobacterium tuberculosis*

6. The OVIVA study (Oral versus Intravenous Antibiotics for Bone and Joint Infection) investigated if oral antibiotic

therapy is noninferior to intravenous antibiotic therapy.[7] Based on the results of this study, would it be appropriate for CJ to receive oral antibiotics?
   A. Yes
   B. No

7. Which of the following oral antibiotic regimens performed worst in the OVIVA study?
   A. Penicillins
   B. Quinolones
   C. Tetracyclines
   D. Macrolides

8. Which of the following selections accurately ranks antibiotics in the order of bioavailability? Rank is from highest to lowest.
   A. Levofloxacin > Azithromycin > Amoxicillin
   B. Doxycycline > Ampicillin > Penicillin
   C. Clarithromycin > Tetracycline > Moxifloxacin
   D. Minocycline > Amoxicillin > Ciprofloxacin

9. Culture and susceptibility results from CJ's bone biopsy have identified methicillin-sensitive *Staphylococcus aureus* (MSSA). CJ is prescribed ceftriaxone 2 g IV q24h. What is the recommended antibiotic duration as per the IDSA Vertebral Osteomyelitis Guidelines?
   A. 4 weeks
   B. 6 weeks
   C. 8 weeks
   D. 12 weeks

10. When should CJ have his ESR and CRP repeated to monitor his response to treatment?
   A. Never, there is no utility in ESR and CRP as monitoring parameters
   B. Daily
   C. Weekly
   D. After 4 weeks of antibiotic therapy

ANSWERS

1. **Explanation:** The correct answer is C. Poor dentition is noted in the physical exam. The three pathways of osteomyelitis are hematogenous spread (through a blood stream infection), direct inoculation from trauma, or contiguous spread from adjacent skin infection. Hematogenous spread is the most common cause and adults with degenerative disc disease are at a higher risk. A systematic review of clinical characteristics of pyogenic (bacterial) vertebral osteomyelitis found that the most common source was the urinary tract, followed by skin infections, intravenous catheters, respiratory, gastrointestinal, or oral infection.[1] Choices A, B, and D are incorrect because CJ has no evidence of skin infection (erythema, edema, warmth), IV drug use (visible tracks or injection site lesions), or symptoms of diverticulitis on physical exam.

2. **Explanation:** The correct answer is B. The major clinical manifestation of vertebral osteomyelitis is back pain.

A patient's pain is typically localized to the infected disc space area and is exacerbated by physical activity or percussion to the affected area. Answer A is incorrect because CJ did not have a fever (temperature ≥38°C). Answer C is incorrect because elevated ESR and CRP are associated with a diagnosis of osteomyelitis but are signs not symptoms. Answer D is incorrect because CJ is not hemodynamically unstable.

3. **Explanation:** The correct answer is D. A study of 173 with a diagnosis of vertebral osteomyelitis found no difference in microbial yield between patients who received antibiotics before or after a biopsy.[2] One study found that a duration of antibiotic of 4 or more days was a risk factor for negative cultures.[3]

4. **Explanation:** The correct answer is C. The IDSA Native Vertebral Osteomyelitis Guidelines recommend delaying antibiotics until a microbiological diagnosis is made for patients with normal and stable neurologic examination and stable hemodynamic.[4] In patients with hemodynamic instability, sepsis, septic shock, or severe or progressive neurologic symptoms, the guidelines suggest initiating empiric antibiotics in conjunction with getting a microbiologic diagnosis. Of note, both recommendations are weak and supported by low quality evidence. In a small study of nondrug users, blood cultures were positive in 72% of patients and can aid in the microbiologic diagnosis in patients with vertebral osteomyelitis.[5]

5. **Explanation:** The correct answer is B. Most patients have monomicrobial infections. The most common cause of vertebral osteomyelitis is *Staphylococcus aureus*. A study in which 101 patients with an identified organism found that methicillin-sensitive *Staphylococcus aureus* (MSSA) was the most prevalent (63%).[6] Gram-positive pathogens (staphylococci and streptococci) accounted for 87% of cultured pathogens compared to 7% for gram-negative bacteria. *Mycobacterium tuberculosis* (MTB) can also cause vertebral osteomyelitis. Unlike pyogenic vertebral osteomyelitis, MTB infections are more subacute and diagnosis is often not made until 4 to 6 months after symptom onset.

6. **Explanation:** The correct answer is A. The OVIVA study included 39 patients with acute or chronic vertebral osteomyelitis.[7] Important exclusion criteria include patients with *Staphylococcus aureus* bloodstream infections and/or endocarditis. The OVIVA study results revealed that treatment failure at 1 year occurred in 15% (74/506) of patients in the IV group and 13% (67/509) in the PO group. These results demonstrated that that PO antibiotics were noninferior to IV antibiotics for the treatment of bone and joint infections.

7. **Explanation:** The correct answer is A. The OVIVA study did not seek to compare specific antibiotic regimens or to stipulate which agents should or should not be used.[7] However, as per Figure S2 from the Supplementary Appendix patients treated with oral penicillins

had a higher numerical, but not statistical, failure rate than patients treated with quinolones, tetracyclines, or macrolides.

	Failure, *n* (%)	No Failure, *n* (%)	Odds Ratio (95% CI)
Penicillins	17/57	9/48	1.6 (0.7–3.9)
Quinolones	20/189	26/179	0.7 (0.4–1.4)
Tetracyclines	7/40	7/30	0.8 (0.2–2.4)
Macrolides	5/53	6/44	0.7 (0.2–2.4)

8. **Explanation:** The correct answer is D. One of the potential reasons suggested for the difference in outcomes among antibiotic classes in the OVIVA study is the differences in bioavailability. While penicillin antibiotics have lower bioavailability as a class than quinolones or tetracyclines, they are higher than macrolides. Dosing frequency is higher among penicillins and may lead to higher failure rates. Of note, adherence rates between the IV and PO groups were similar. Another difference between antibiotics is bone penetration which may impact cure rates.[8] While the OVIVA trial is an important trial and demonstrated that PO antibiotics can safely be used to treat bone and joint infections, we are still in need of more information about specific antibiotics and dosing regimens.

Antibiotic	Bioavailability[9]	Frequency	Bone concentration[8] (mcg/g)
Penicillin VK	60%	4 × daily	unknown
Ampicillin	50%	4 × daily	12–20
Amoxicillin	77–80%	2–3 × daily	15–20
Ciprofloxacin	60–80%	2 × daily	0.7–1.4
Moxifloxacin	90%	1 × daily	1.3–1.9
Levofloxacin	99%	1 × daily	3–6
Tetracycline	85%	4 × daily	unknown
Doxycycline	95%	2 × daily	0.1–2.6
Minocycline	95%	2 × daily	0.4–0.9
Azithromycin	38%	1 × daily	1.9
Clarithromycin	55%	2 × daily	unknown

9. **Explanation:** The correct answer is B. The IDSA Vertebral Osteomyelitis Guidelines suggest 6 weeks of antibiotics for all bacterial infections except *Salmonella* species for which recommendations are 6 to 8 weeks of antibiotics.[4] A randomized trial of patients with pyogenic vertebral osteomyelitis compared outcomes between 6 and 12 weeks of antibiotics.[10] Clinical cure at 1 year was 91% in both the 6- and 12-week treatment groups. Nearly half of the patients in this trial received an oral fluoroquinolone and rifampicin. Contrary to these results, the median duration of antibiotics in the OVIVA study is 11 weeks in the IV group and 10 weeks in the PO group.[7]

10. **Explanation:** The correct answer is C. The IDSA Vertebral Osteomyelitis Guidelines suggest monitoring systemic inflammatory markers (ESR and/or CRP) after approximately 4 weeks of antibiotic therapy.[4] Monitoring ESR and CRP may help identify patients at greater risk for treatment failure. Patients with a 50% reduction in ESR after 4 weeks rarely develop treatment failure.[11] Of note, most patients who do not experience a significant drop in systemic inflammatory markers still have successful outcomes.

REFERENCES

1. Mylona E, Samarkos M, Kakalou E, Fanourgiakis P, Skoutelis A. Pyogenic vertebral osteomyelitis: a systematic review of clinical characteristics. *Semin Arthritis Rheum.* 2009;39(1):10-17.

2. Saravolatz LD, Labalo V, Fishbain J, Szpunar S, Johnson LB. Lack of effect of antibiotics on biopsy culture results in vertebral osteomyelitis. *Diagn Microbiol Infect Dis.* 2018;91(3):273-274.

3. Kim CJ, Song KH, Park WB, et al. Microbiologically and clinically diagnosed vertebral osteomyelitis: impact of prior antibiotic exposure. *Antimicrob Agents Chemother.* 2012;56(4):2122-2124.

4. Berbari EF, Kanj SS, Kowalski TJ, et al. 2015 Infectious Diseases Society of America (IDSA) clinical practice guidelines for the diagnosis and treatment of native vertebral osteomyelitis in adults. *Clin Infect Dis.* 2015;61(6):e26-e46.

5. Nolla JM, Ariza J, Gómez-Vaquero C, et al. Spontaneous pyogenic vertebral osteomyelitis in nondrug users. *Semin Arthritis Rheum.* 2002;31(4):271-278.

6. Chong BSW, Brereton CJ, Gordon A, Davis JS. Epidemiology, microbiological diagnosis, and clinical outcomes in pyogenic vertebral osteomyelitis: a 10-year retrospective cohort study. *Open Forum Infect Dis.* 2018;5(3):ofy037.

7. Li HK, Rombach I, Zambellas R, et al. Oral versus intravenous antibiotics for bone and joint infection. *N Engl J Med.* 2019;380(5):425-436.

8. Spellberg B, Lipsky BA. Systemic antibiotic therapy for chronic osteomyelitis in adults. *Clin Infect Dis.* 2012;54(3):393-407.

9. IBM Micromedex®. *Micromedex Solutions.* Ann Arbor, MI: Truven Health Analytics.

10. Bernard L, Dinh A, Ghout I, et al. Antibiotic treatment for 6 weeks versus 12 weeks in patients with pyogenic vertebral osteomyelitis: an open-label, non-inferiority, randomised, controlled trial. *Lancet.* 2015;385(9971):875-882.

11. Yoon SH, Chung SK, Kim KJ, Kim HJ, Jin YJ, Kim HB. Pyogenic vertebral osteomyelitis: identification of microorganism and laboratory markers used to predict clinical outcome. *Eur Spine J.* 2010;19(4):575-582.

20 Prosthetic Joint Infection

Amelia K. Sofjan

PATIENT PRESENTATION

Chief Complaint

"My right knee hurts really bad."

History of Present Illness

AD is a 66-year-old female who had a right total knee arthroplasty (TKA) and has been experiencing right knee pain that has increased gradually in severity since 2 weeks ago. The pain is persistent and moderate to severe. She also has been having trouble walking around the block. Of note, the right knee is swollen and red. She followed up in clinic with her surgeon yesterday and was told she needed to be admitted to the hospital.

Past Medical History

Obesity, type 2 diabetes, osteoarthritis, hypertension, hyperlipidemia, depression

Surgical History

Right TKA 3 weeks ago, C-section

Family History

Father died at age 62 from a heart attack; mother died at age 70 from breast cancer

Social History

No alcohol, tobacco, or IV drug use; lives at home with her husband; she is retired

Allergies

Septra ("bad rash")

Home Medications

Metformin 1000 mg PO BID
Desvenlafaxine 50 mg PO daily
Ibuprofen 600 mg PO TID PRN
Lisinopril 40 mg PO daily
Hydrochlorothiazide 25 mg PO daily
Simvastatin 80 mg PO daily

Physical Examination

▶ **Vital Signs**

Temp 100°F, P 78, RR 16 breaths per minute, BP 148/92 mm Hg, pO_2 98% on room air, Ht 5′4″, Wt 90.7 kg

▶ **General**

Well-groomed female in moderate distress

▶ **HEENT**

PERRLA, EOMI

▶ **Pulmonary**

Clear to auscultation, no crackles or wheezing

▶ **Cardiovascular**

RRR, no m/r/g

▶ **Abdomen**

Normal BS, abdomen soft and tender

▶ **Neurology**

A&O ×3, CN II-XII grossly intact

▶ **Extremities**

Right knee is edematous and erythematous; knee feels stable but warm to the touch

Laboratory Findings

Na = 140 mEq/L	Hgb = 14.1 g/dL	AST = 20 IU/L
K = 4.3 mEq/L	Hct = 42%	ALT = 24 IU/L
Cl = 102 mEq/L	Plt = 167 × 10^3/mm^3	T Bili = 1.5 mg/dL
CO_2 = 27 mEq/L	WBC = 9 × 10^3/mm^3	Alk Phos = 86 IU/L
BUN = 24 mg/dL		
Scr = 1.01 mg/dL		
Glu = 158 mg/dL		

QUESTIONS

1. Which of the following is the most common organism isolated in PJI?
   A. *Staphylococcus*
   B. *Enterococcus*
   C. *Streptococcus*
   D. Gram-negative bacilli

2. AD's ESR was 40 mm/hr, and CRP was 15 mg/dL. An arthrocentesis (joint aspiration) revealed a leukocyte count of 5,100 cells/μL (88% neutrophils). The synovial fluid aerobic culture is positive for CONS. AD was taken to the operating room for an inspection of her right knee, and the intra-operative note stated purulence surrounding the prosthesis. Which of AD's findings is definitive for PJI?
   A. Elevated ESR and CRP
   B. Elevated leukocyte and neutrophil count of the synovial fluid
   C. Synovial culture positive for CONS
   D. Purulence surrounding the prosthesis

3. The orthopedic surgeon opted for DAIR (debridement, antibiotics, and implant retention) to manage AD's PJI. Is DAIR a reasonable surgical strategy for AD?
   A. Yes, because the synovial leukocyte and neutrophil count were not extremely high
   B. Yes, because the prosthesis was implanted 3 weeks ago
   C. No, because her symptoms have lasted for 2 weeks
   D. No, because her synovial fluid is positive for CONS

4. AD's pre-operative synovial fluid and 2 intra-operative cultures are growing CONS with the following susceptibility report: oxacillin (R), vancomycin (S), tetracycline (S), TMP/SMX (S), clindamycin (R), rifampin (S), linezolid (S), ciprofloxacin (S), daptomycin (S). Which of the following is the preferred initial antibiotic therapy for AD? AD is willing to switch her non-infective drugs if needed except her antidepressant.
   A. Vancomycin
   B. Rifampin
   C. Vancomycin plus rifampin
   D. Linezolid
   E. Daptomycin

5. AD was initiated on vancomycin plus rifampin for 4 weeks and is now being transitioned to an all oral regimen. Which of the following is the most optimal recommendation?
   A. Ciprofloxacin 750 mg PO BID
   B. Doxycycline 100 mg PO BID
   C. Levofloxacin 250 mg PO daily + rifampin 300 mg PO BID
   D. Ciprofloxacin 750 mg PO BID + rifampin 300 mg PO BID

6. Which of the following is the recommended total antibiotic treatment duration for AD?
   A. 4 to 6 weeks
   B. 3 to 6 months
   C. 7 to 11 months
   D. 12 to 24 months

7. Two years later, AD is diagnosed with another episode of staphylococcal PJI and will undergo a 2-stage exchange. How is the antibiotic treatment for this 2-stage exchange similar or different compared to the treatment for DAIR that AD received initially?
   A. AD will need rifampin as part of combination therapy just like in DAIR
   B. AD will need 3–6 months of antibiotic therapy just like in DAIR
   C. AD will need pathogen-specific therapy up until the day of the reimplantation
   D. AD will need pathogen-specific therapy for 4 to 6 weeks

ANSWERS

1. **Explanation:** The correct answer is A. Choices B, C, and D are incorrect because the most common organisms isolated in PJI are coagulase-negative *Staphylococcus* (CONS) and *Staphylococcus aureus* (50% to 60%), followed by *Enterococcus* and *Streptococcus* (10%). Gram-negative bacilli are uncommon, and fungal and atypical bacteria have been typically isolated in patients with malignancy, autoimmune or immunocompromising conditions, or prolonged antibiotic use.[1]

2. **Explanation:** The correct answer is D. Choice A is incorrect because elevated ESR and CRP are supportive of a PJI diagnosis but nonspecific. Choice B is incorrect because elevated leukocyte and neutrophil count have good sensitivity and specificity for PJI but are not definitive. Choice C is incorrect because one culture positive for a common skin flora such as CONS is not definitive for PJI and must be interpreted in the context of other findings. However, two cultures (both intra-operative or one pre-operative and one intra-operative) growing the same organism is definitive for PJI. Purulence surrounding the prosthesis in the absence of other etiology, a sinus tract that communicates with the prosthesis, or acute inflammation in histopathological exam is definitive for PJI.[1,2]

3. **Explanation:** The correct answer is B. Please see table for the different types of surgical options and their respective patient candidates.[2] Synovial leukocyte and neutrophil count are not determinants of surgical management (rules out choice A). Choice C is incorrect because AD's symptoms lasted <3 weeks, which makes her a good candidate for DAIR. Choice D is incorrect because CONS is not virulent and typically not multidrug resistant, making DAIR a reasonable strategy. PJIs due to more virulent organisms, such as *S. aureus*, have been associated with increased rates of DAIR failure, and it may be worse with methicillin-resistant *S. aureus* (MRSA).[3] However, a recent study did not find this association.[4] DAIR can still be appropriate for

MRSA PJIs depending on other patient-specific factors as listed in the table.

Surgical management of PJI: description of procedure and patient candidates

Debridement, antibiotics, and implant retention (DAIR)
Debridement, exchange of modular components, and prolonged antibiotic therapy

- Symptom duration <3 weeks or prosthesis implantation within past 30 days PLUS well-fixed prosthesis, no sinus tract, and organism susceptible to oral antibiotic agents
- Elderly patients with comorbidities unable to do 1- or 2-stage exchange

1-stage exchange
Removal of implant, debridement, and implantation of new prosthesis all in the same surgery

- Typically done in Europe

2-stage exchange
Removal of implant, debridement ± placement of antibiotic-impregnated spacer, antibiotic therapy (1st surgery), then spacer exchange or prosthesis reimplantation (2nd surgery)

- Commonly used in the United States if medically stable and able to undergo multiple surgeries

Permanent resection arthroplasty
Removal of implant with or without arthrodesis (joint fusion) or limb amputation

- Non-ambulatory, multiple comorbidities, or minimal bone stock or soft tissue coverage
- Multidrug-resistant organisms or refractory/relapsing infection despite all efforts
- Failed prior 2-stage exchange and infection risk after reimplantation is unacceptable

Source: Data from Osmon DR, Berbari EF, Berendt AR, et al. Diagnosis and management of prosthetic joint infection. *Clin Infect Dis.* 2013;56:e1–e25.

4. **Explanation:** The correct answer is C. The initial treatment of choice following DAIR for oxacillin-resistant staphylococcal PJI is vancomycin plus rifampin (if the staphylococcus is susceptible to rifampin and rifampin can be used safely) for 2 to 6 weeks.[2] Vancomycin is preferred due to established clinical experience but requires therapeutic drug monitoring and can cause nephrotoxicity and leukopenia. Rifampin is used for staphylococcal PJI managed by DAIR because of its activity against biofilm organisms which form in the presence of a foreign body. Rifampin should always be used in combination due to a high rate of resistance emergence if used alone (rules out choice B). Two observational studies and a randomized controlled trial of patients with staphylococcal PJI, in which 21% to 44% of patients had CONS (the rest had *S. aureus*), showed the benefit of rifampin combination.[5–7] Although the case for adding rifampin is stronger for *S. aureus* PJI, rifampin should be added for CONS PJI if

benefits outweigh the risks. Rifampin can cause hepatotoxicity and interacts with many drugs including AD's simvastatin. In this case the drug can be switched to another statin, but sometimes it may not be feasible to modify the interacting medication, thus precluding rifampin use. Linezolid (choice D) has a success rate of about 80% but is an alternative agent due to less clinical experience and risk of thrombocytopenia, peripheral neuropathy, and optic neuritis with prolonged use.[3,8] Linezolid is also a weak monoamine-oxidase inhibitor and interacts with desvenlafaxine, putting AD at risk for serotonin syndrome, a rare but serious event.[9] Daptomycin (choice E) dosed at about 6 to 8 mg/kg/d has a success rate ranging from 58% to 88% but is currently an alternative agent due to less clinical experience, although more data have been published recently.[3,10,11] Daptomycin has been used as salvage therapy or when vancomycin cannot be used due to allergy or toxicities. It can cause elevated CPK, myopathy, and rarely rhabdomyolysis. Twice weekly CPK monitoring is prudent in patients on concomitant statin and daptomycin to minimize these adverse effects.

5. **Explanation:** The correct answer is D. Because the implant is retained, rifampin should be continued for its activity against biofilm organisms in staphylococcal PJI. The treatment of choice following IV therapy plus rifampin is an oral agent plus rifampin (rules out choices A and B).[2,5–7] Levofloxacin or ciprofloxacin is a first-line oral agent for staphylococcal PJI based on good efficacy data.[6,12] Choice C is incorrect because levofloxacin should be dosed at 750 mg PO daily.[12]

6. **Explanation:** The correct answer is B. IDSA guidelines recommend 6 months for TKA and 3 months for total hip arthroplasty (THA) based on older studies.[2,5–7] However, a recent observational study of *S. aureus* PJI managed with DAIR reported a mean ± SD treatment duration of 12.6 ± 7 weeks, which was similar for TKA and THA.[13] In this study, longer treatment duration was independently associated with success at 2 years. Overall the evidence suggests TKA may be potentially treated as short as 3 months like THA and up to 6 months. Lastly, a recent randomized trial of patients with acute staphylococcal PJI managed with DAIR showed no difference in cure rates between 8 weeks vs 3 months or 6 months of treatment duration for THA or TKA, respectively. However, the trial had a small sample size and was not adequately powered; hence, the benefit of antibiotics beyond 8 weeks cannot be ruled out.[12] Nevertheless, shorter treatment duration should be evaluated in larger future trials. Current evidence does not support choice A, C, or D.

7. **Explanation:** The correct answer is D. The recommended medical management in patients undergoing a 2-stage exchange is 4 to 6 weeks of pathogen-specific intravenous or highly bioavailable oral antibiotic therapy. Because the implant is removed in a 2-stage exchange, rifampin is not generally recommended and the treatment duration is

shorter (4 to 6 weeks) than that of DAIR (rules out choices A and B). In contrast, rifampin and prolonged antibiotic therapy are necessary in patients with staphylococcal PJI undergoing DAIR because the implant is retained. Choice C is incorrect because after a patient receives 4 to 6 weeks of antibiotic therapy, antibiotics should be stopped for 2 to 4 weeks prior to reimplantation to optimize the diagnostic yield of cultures during reimplantation.[2]

REFERENCES

1. Abad CL, Haleem A. Prosthetic joint infections. *Curr Infect Dis Rep.* 2018;20:15.
2. Osmon DR, Berbari EF, Berendt AR, et al. Diagnosis and management of prosthetic joint infection. *Clin Infect Dis.* 2013;56:e1-e25.
3. Salgado CD, Dash S, Cantey JR, Marculescu CE. Higher risk of failure of methicillin-resistant *Staphylococcus aureus* prosthetic joint infections. *Clin Orthop Relat Res.* 2007;461:48-53.
4. Fink B, Schuster P, Schwenninger C, Frommelt L, Oremek DA. A standardized regimen for the treatment of acute postoperative infections and acute hematogenous infections associated with hip and knee arthroplasties. *J Arthroplast.* 2017;32(4):1255-1261.
5. Widmer AF, Gaechter A, Ochsner PE, Zimmerli W. Antimicrobial treatment of orthopedic implant-related infections with rifampin combinations. *Clin Infect Dis.* 1992;14:1251-1253.
6. Zimmerli W, Widmer AF, Blatter M. Role of rifampin for treatment of orthopedic-implant related staphylococcal infections: a randomized controlled trial. *JAMA.* 1998;279:1537-1541.
7. Peel TN, Buising KL, Dowsey MM, et al. Outcome of debridement and retention in prosthetic joint infections by methicillin-resistant staphylococci, with special reference to rifampin and fusidic acid combination therapy. *Antimicrob Agents Chemother.* 2013;57:350-355.
8. Morata L, Tornero E, Martínez-Pastor JC, García-Ramiro S, Mensa J, Soriano A. Clinical experience with linezolid for the treatment of orthopaedic implant infections. *J Antimicrob Chemother.* 2014;69(suppl 1):i47-i52.
9. Karkow DC, Kauer JF, Ernst EJ. Incidence of serotonin syndrome with combined use of linezolid and serotonin reuptake inhibitors compared with linezolid monotherapy. *J Clin Psychopharmacol.* 2017;37(5):518-523.
10. Chang YJ, Lee MS, Lee CH, Lin PC, Kuo FC. Daptomycin treatment in patients with resistant staphylococcal periprosthetic joint infection. *BMC Infect Dis.* 2017;17:736.
11. Malizos K, Sarma J, Seaton RA, et al. Daptomycin for the treatment of osteomyelitis and orthopaedic device infections: real-world clinical experience from a European registry. *Eur J Clin Microbiol Infect Dis.* 2016;35:111-118.
12. Lora-Tamayo J, Euba G, Cobo J, et al. Short- versus long-duration levofloxacin plus rifampicin for acute staphylococcal prosthetic joint infection managed with implant retention: a randomized clinical trial. *Int J Antimicrob Agents.* 2016;48:310-316.
13. Lesens O, Ferry T, Forestier E, et al. Should we expand the indications for the DAIR (debridement, antibiotic therapy, and implant retention) procedure for *Staphylococcus aureus* prosthetic joint infections? A multicenter retrospective study. *Eur J Clin Microbiol Infect Dis.* 2018;37:1949-1956.

21 Intra-Abdominal Infections

Jamie L. Wagner

PATIENT PRESENTATION

Chief Complaint
"My belly keeps filling with fluid, and I don't feel well."

History of Present Illness
SB is a 49-year-old female with a PMH of HCV who presented with complaints of sharp, constant abdominal pain and swelling.

Past Medical History

▶ **Childhood Illnesses**

Measles at age 5, recurrent OM

▶ **Travel**

Recent trip to Arizona

▶ **Habits**

+ EtOH, (–) tobacco, (–) illicits

▶ **Immunizations**

Up-to-date on all childhood immunizations

▶ **Surgical History**

Two pins in R great toe s/p bunion repair

▶ **Family History**

Mother: MI, DM2, dyslipidemia, obesity
Father: DM2, obesity, deceased at age 50

▶ **Social History**

SB currently lives with her mother. She works a full-time job as a teller at the local credit union.

▶ **Allergies**

NKDA

▶ **Home Medications**

None

Physical Examination

▶ **General Appearance**

Cachectic appearing female in NAD, supine in bed

▶ **Vital Signs**

Temp 101.5°F, HR 80, BP 108/72, RR 16 breaths per minute, SpO_2 98% RA, Ht 5'4", Wt 46 kg

▶ **Skin, Hair, and Nails**

Jaundice, no rashes or bruises

▶ **HEENT**

AT, bitemporal wasting, PERRL b/l, no ptosis, + scleral icterus, nares patent, MMM

▶ **Neck**

Supple, NROM, + JVD

▶ **Chest and Lungs**

CtAB, no w/r/r

▶ **Heart**

RRR, no m/r/g, severe pitting edema to level of abdomen

▶ **Abdomen**

Taut, distended, fluid wave, midline large hernia, caput medusae, RUQ guarding, hypoactive bs, massive ascites

▶ **Extremities**

3+ pitting edema BLLE

▶ **Neurologic**

Sensation intact, CN II-XII intact, strength 5/5 in UE and LE, + asterixis, + ataxia

▶ **Psychiatric**

Appears confused, somnolent

Laboratory Findings

Chemistry, Coags, CBC

Sodium (136–146) mmol/L	Potassium (3.5–5.1) mmol/L	Chloride (98–108) mmol/L	CO$_2$ (20–30) mmol/L	BUN (7–17) mg/dL	Creatinine (0.5–1.2) mg/dL	Glucose (74–106) mg/dL	Calcium (8.4–10.2) mg/dL
122	4.1	96	20	20	1.87	86	9.1
T. Protein (6.6-8.7) g/dL	Albumin (3.5–5.5) g/dL	T. Bili (0–1) mg/dL	D. Bili (0–0.3) mg/dL	I. Bili (0–1.1) mg/dL	Alk Phos (40–129) U/L	AST (0–40) U/L	ALT (0–41) U/L
6.2	2.3	18.6	10.5	8.1	263	108	52
PT (11–13.5) sec	INR (<1.1)	Ammonia (15–45) mcg/dL	WBC (4.0–11.0) th/cmm	RBC (4.5–5.4) m/cmm	Hgb (12.5–15.5) g/dL	Hct (39.0–45.0) %	Platelets (130–400) th/cmm
17.8	1.84	153	13.5	4.5	12.1	36.5	42

CT Abdomen

▸ *ABDOMEN*

Nodular contour of the liver which demonstrates diffuse low attenuation of the hepatic parenchyma. No gallbladder wall thickening and/or presence of pericholecystic fluid. No biliary dilatation. There is presence of portosystemic varices within the anterior abdominal wall and upper abdomen. Splenomegaly with findings of portal venous hypertension. Large amount of ascites present.

▸ *IMPRESSION*

Diffuse low-attenuation of the hepatic parenchyma with nodular contour favoring steatosis/cirrhosis. Splenomegaly and extensive varices with findings of portal venous hypertension.

▸ *Cultures*

Blood Cx pending

QUESTIONS

1. Which laboratory test(s) help identify a patient with spontaneous bacterial peritonitis?
   A. Positive blood culture
   B. Ascitic cell count and differential
   C. Ascitic albumin
   D. Serum ammonia

2. What is a sign or symptom of spontaneous bacterial peritonitis in SB?
   A. Demonstration of abdominal pain
   B. Presence of portosystemic varices
   C. Explainable encephalopathy
   D. All of the above

3. SB's ascitic fluid analysis revealed PMN count of 729 cells/mm³. The diagnosis of spontaneous bacterial peritonitis is made. Which empirical therapy is most appropriate for SB?
   A. Cefazolin
   B. Piperacillin/tazobactam

   C. Vancomycin
   D. Ceftriaxone

4. The preliminary ascitic fluid Gram stain resulted in gram (–) bacilli. Which of the following pathogens is most likely to be cultured?
   A. *Salmonella enterica*
   B. *Citrobacter freundii*
   C. *Klebsiella pneumoniae*
   D. *Pseudomonas putida*

5. *Escherichia coli* was isolated from the ascitic fluid culture. How long would you treat SB?
   A. 3 days
   B. 5 days
   C. 7 days
   D. 10 days

6. SB is discharged from the hospital with prophylaxis against another episode of SBP. What is the recommended antibiotic for SBP prophylaxis in a non-hospitalized patient?
   A. Ciprofloxacin 500 mg PO daily
   B. Doxycycline 100 mg PO daily
   C. Amoxicillin 875 mg PO daily
   D. Cefdinir 300 mg PO daily

7. SB is readmitted to the hospital 3 weeks later with a variceal hemorrhage. Which of the following should be started to provide prophylaxis for SBP for this admission?
   A. Oral trimethoprim/sulfamethoxazole
   B. Oral ciprofloxacin
   C. IV ceftriaxone
   D. IV ampicillin

8. SB should receive long-term prophylaxis against SBP based upon which of the following risk factors?
   A. Ascitic fluid total protein <1.5 g/dL
   B. Previous variceal hemorrhage
   C. Previous SBP episode
   D. All of the above

ANSWERS

1. **Explanation:** The correct answer is B. Answer A is incorrect because infection within the peritoneum does not always infiltrate the bloodstream; therefore, ascitic fluid cultures would be more accurate and appropriate. Answer C is incorrect because ascitic albumin is used to help diagnose the presence of portal hypertension, not spontaneous bacterial peritonitis. Answer D is incorrect because serum ammonia is used to help diagnose hepatic encephalopathy, not spontaneous bacterial peritonitis. Answer B is correct because spontaneous bacterial peritonitis (eg, primary peritonitis) is diagnosed by an elevated ascitic fluid absolute polymorphonuclear leukocyte (PMNs) $\geq$250 cells/mm^3 without an evident intra-abdominal, surgically treatable infection.[1]

2. **Explanation:** The correct answer is A. Answer B is incorrect because the presence of varices is not indicative of SBP, but rather, portal hypertension. Answer C is incorrect because SBP is related to unexplainable encephalopathy (eg, ammonia within normal limits) instead of explainable encephalopathy. Answer A is correct because pain within the abdominal cavity in a patient with ascites, in addition to fever and unexplained encephalopathy, are indicators that an infection is most likely present and empiric therapy should be started.[1]

3. **Explanation:** The correct answer is D. Answer A is incorrect because the spectrum of activity is not reliable to provide coverage against all the suspected gram-negative pathogens (eg, Enterobacteriaceae). Answer B is incorrect because the spectrum of activity is unnecessarily broad for treating the suspected gram-negative pathogens by providing coverage against anaerobes and *Pseudomonas aeruginosa*. Answer C is incorrect because no gram-negative coverage is provided. Answer D is correct because the spectrum of activity of ceftriaxone can cover 95% of the suspected infecting organisms.[1]

4. **Explanation:** The correct answer is C. Answer C is correct because *K. pneumoniae* is one of the 3 most common isolates, which also include *E. coli* and *S. pneumoniae*. Answers A, B, and D are all possible options for causing SBP; however, the most commonly isolated pathogen out of the answer choices provided is answer C.[1]

5. **Explanation:** The correct answer is B. According to the guidelines,[1] a randomized controlled trial of 100 patients demonstrated that 5 days of therapy was as effective as 10 days of therapy for treatment of SBP.[2] Therefore, answers A, C, and D are incorrect.

6. **Explanation:** The correct answer is A. Answers B, C, and D are incorrect because spectrum of activity and/or probability for adequate target attainment into ascitic fluid are not sufficient for prophylaxis. Answer A is correct based upon previous data with norfloxacin success rates in preventing SBP in patients who have already experienced at least 1 episode.[3] Routine prophylaxis for gut decontamination in cirrhosis patients does not select for resistant bacteria.[4]

7. **Explanation:** The correct answer is C. While PO trimethoprim/sulfamethoxazole and PO ciprofloxacin can be used to prevent SBP on an outpatient basis, during an acute variceal bleed, IV therapy is recommended.[1] Therefore, answers A and B are incorrect. Answer D is incorrect because the spectrum of activity is not adequate to cover all the suspected pathogens and has been proven to be inferior to third-generation cephalosporins.[5] Answer C is correct because IV ceftriaxone for 7 days has demonstrated efficacy in preventing SBP in patients with cirrhosis and GI-related hemorrhages.[5]

8. **Explanation:** The correct answer is D. According to the guidelines, answers A, B, and C were identified as risk factors most closely associated with subsequent episodes of SBP. Other patient characteristics (eg, number of previous SBP episodes, age, sex, etiology of cirrhosis, liver function tests, previous treatment for SBP, previously isolated organisms) are not used to guide prescribing prophylaxis, as this would lead to a more liberal use of antibiotics, eventually leading to colonization and subsequent infection by resistant flora.[1,6]

REFERENCES

1. Runyon BA. Management of adult patients with ascites due to cirrhosis: update 2012. *Hepatology*. 2013;57(4):1-27. Available at https://www.aasld.org/sites/default/files/2019-06/AASLDPracticeGuidelineAsciteDuetoCirrhosisUpdate2012Edition4_.pdf.

2. Runyon BA, McHutchison JG, Antillon MR, Akriviadis EA, Montano A. Short-course vs long-course antibiotic treatment of spontaneous bacterial peritonitis: a randomized controlled trial of 100 patients. *Gastroenterology*. 1991;100:1737-1742.

3. Gines P, Rimola A, Planas R, Vargas V, Marco F, Almela M, et al. Norfloxacin prevents spontaneous bacterial peritonitis recurrence in cirrhosis: results of a double-blind, placebo-controlled trial. *Hepatology*. 1990;12:716-724.

4. Fernandez J, Acevedo J, Castro M, Garcia O, Rodriquez de Lope C, Roca D, et al. Prevalence and risk factors of infections by resistant bacteria in cirrhosis: a prospective study. *Hepatology*. 2012;55:1551-1561.

5. Felisart J, Rimola A, Arroyo V, Perez-Ayuso RM, Quintero E, Gines P, et al. Randomized comparative study of efficacy and nephrotoxicity of ampicillin plus tobramycin versus cefotaxime in cirrhotics with severe infections. *Hepatology*. 1985;5:457-462.

6. Tító L, Rimola A, Ginés P, Llach J, Arroyo V, Rodés J. Recurrence of spontaneous bacterial peritonitis in cirrhosis: frequency and predictive factors. *Hepatology*. 1988;8:27-31.

22 *Clostridioides difficile* Infection

Rebecca L. Dunn   Jonathan C. Cho

PATIENT PRESENTATION

Chief Complaint

Watery diarrhea

History of Present Illness

AH is a 52-year-old Caucasian male with a recent history of hospitalization for cellulitis. He presents to the emergency department with watery diarrhea. He reports approximately 5 unformed stools per day over the last 3 days. He also complains of fever, chills, abdominal cramping, and general fatigue. He states that he was admitted to the hospital 10 days prior for cellulitis of the right knee and was treated with clindamycin. He was discharged, after a 2-day admission, on 5 additional days of clindamycin therapy.

Past Medical History

T2DM, diabetic neuropathy, HTN, HLD, chronic venous stasis, obesity, GERD, cellulitis (resolved)

Family History

Father with T2DM, obesity, and deceased at age 71 secondary to a myocardial infarction. Mother with HTN (living). Sibling with T2DM, HTN (living)

Social History

Tobacco 1/4 ppd × 45 years (quit 8 years prior); 1 (12 oz) beer per day. No illicit drug use

Allergies

Penicillin (swelling of the face)

Home Medications

Metformin 1000 mg PO BID
Glipizide XL 10 mg PO daily
Pregabalin 100 mg PO TID
Lisinopril/HCTZ 20 mg/12.5 mg, 2 tablets PO daily
Amlodipine/atorvastatin 10 mg/80 mg PO daily
ASA 81 mg PO daily
Omeprazole 20 mg PO daily
Clindamycin 450 mg PO QID (recently completed a 7-day course of therapy)

Physical Examination

▸ *Vital Signs*

Temp 102.7°F, P 88, RR 18 breaths per minute, BP 158/88 mm Hg, pO$_2$ 94%, Ht 5′10″, Wt 141 kg

▸ *General*

Mild distress, obese

▸ *HEENT*

Normocephalic, atraumatic, PERRLA, EOMI, pink/moist mucous membranes and conjunctiva, no headache, no neck stiffness/pain, no photophobia

▸ *Pulmonary*

CTAB

▸ *Cardiovascular*

NSR, no m/r/g, DOE

▸ *Abdomen*

Soft, non-distended, mildly tender to palpation, positive guarding, bowel sounds hyperactive

▸ *Genitourinary*

Normal male genitalia, no complaints of dysuria or hematuria

▸ *Neurology*

A&O ×3, cranial nerves intact

▸ *Extremities*

Normal range of motion, no edema, changes consistent with venous stasis

Emergency Department Labs

Na = 140 mEq/L	Hgb = 14.6 g/dL	AST = 36 IU/L
K = 4.2 mEq/L	Hct = 42%	ALT = 28 IU/L
Cl = 106 mEq/L	Plt = 160 × 10³/mm³	Alk Phos = 69 IU/L
CO$_2$ = 26 mEq/L	WBC = 18.1 × 10³/mm³	Albumin = 4.2 g/dL
BUN = 21 mg/dL	Neutros = 75%	T Bili = 1.7 mg/dL
SCr = 1.7 mg/dL	Bands = 9%	Mg = 2.0 mg/dL
Glu = 209 mg/dL	Lymphs = 15%	Phos = 4.1 mg/dL
	Monos = 1%	Ca = 9.8 mg/dL

▸ *C. difficile Toxin Enzyme Immunoassay (EIA)*

A/B toxin assay positive

► **Blood Cultures**

Pending

► **Urine Cultures**

Pending

► **Fecal Occult Blood Test (FOBT)**

Negative

QUESTIONS

1. According to the clinical practice guidelines by the Infectious Diseases Society of America (IDSA) and Society for Healthcare Epidemiology of America (SHEA), how is AH's *Clostridioides difficile* infection (CDI) defined?
   A. Community-associated (CA) CDI
   B. Community-onset, health care facility-associated (CO-HCFA) CDI
   C. Health care facility–onset (HO) CDI
   D. Recurrent CDI

2. What risk factors does AH have for the development of CDI? (select all that apply)
   A. Age (52 years old)
   B. Serum creatinine (1.7 mg/dL)
   C. Recent antibiotic exposure
   D. Recent hospitalization

3. What finding qualifies AH for *C. difficile* testing?
   A. 5 unformed bowel movements per day
   B. PPI use
   C. Recent antibiotic exposure
   D. Recent hospitalization

4. What laboratory methods are available to diagnose patients with suspected CDI?
   A. Stool toxin test (toxin A and B enzyme immunoassay)
   B. Glutamate dehydrogenase (GDH) enzyme immunoassay
   C. Nucleic acid amplification test (NAAT)
   D. All of the above

5. What is the most appropriate treatment for AH?
   A. Vancomycin 125 mg PO QID for 10 days
   B. Metronidazole 500 mg PO TID for 10 days
   C. Fecal microbiota transplantation
   D. Vancomycin 500 mg PO QID + metronidazole 500 mg IV Q8H

6. What follow-up and monitoring is most appropriate for AH?
   A. Resolution of clinical signs and symptoms
   B. Repeat NAAT
   C. Stool toxin test (toxin A and B enzyme immunoassay)
   D. Glutamate dehydrogenase (GDH) enzyme immunoassay

7. When providing care for patients with CDI, what infection prevention and control measures should be used? (select all that apply)
   A. Donning of gloves and gowns by health care providers
   B. Handwashing with soap and water
   C. Hand antisepsis with alcohol-based products
   D. Isolation of asymptomatic carriers of *C. difficile*
   E. Antibiotic stewardship

ANSWERS

1. **Explanation:** The correct answer is B. To increase comparability of CDI cases and improve surveillance efforts between clinical settings, the use of standardized definitions is recommended. CDI can be defined in several ways. Community-associated (CA) cases are those occurring in patients with no inpatient stay in the previous 12 weeks. Community-onset health care facility–associated (CO-HCFA) cases are of CDI occurring within 28 days after discharge from a health care facility. Due to AH's recent hospital admission, his episode most closely matches this definition. Health care facility-onset (HO) CDI are cases occurring >3 days after admission to a health care facility. Finally, recurrent CDI is defined as an episode with positive symptoms and diagnostic assay following a confirmed episode within the previous 2–8 weeks.[1]

2. **Explanation:** The correct answers are C and D. *C. difficile* is the most common cause of infectious diarrhea in health care settings, and represents a significant burden on the health care system and affected individuals. Although the body of associative risk factors is not well defined, understanding risk factors can aid in prevention and diagnosis. The most important risk factor for the development of CDI is exposure to antibiotics. Antibiotics suppress normal bowel flora, creating an environment for *C. difficile* to grow. Third- and fourth-generation cephalosporins, fluoroquinolones, carbapenems, and clindamycin carry the highest risk. However, almost all antibiotics have been implicated. Multiple antibiotics and duration of exposure also compound the risk of CDI. The risk increases during therapy and for approximately 3 months following therapy. AH has just completed a course of clindamycin; therefore, this is his primary risk factor, making answer C appropriate. Additionally, AH has recently been discharged from the hospital, which increases his risk further (the longer the duration of hospitalization the higher the risk). While renal dysfunction is a risk for complicated disease, it is not a risk factor for the development of CDI on its own (rules out option B). Finally, AH's age is not considered of advanced age (rules out option A). Other risk factors in the development of CDI include chemotherapy, human immunodeficiency virus, manipulation or surgery of the gastrointestinal tract, inflammatory bowel disease, immunosuppression, and renal failure. Use of proton pump inhibitors (PPIs) has also been implicated. While the risk associated with PPIs is a source of debate, they may decrease the protective effects of stomach acid, allowing *C. difficile* to take hold.[1]

3. **Explanation:** The correct answer is A. Clinically, CDI should be suspected in those with new-onset diarrhea,

with current or recent antimicrobial use. However, the evidence surrounding appropriate testing for CDI is weak. According to the IDSA/SHEA practice guidelines, patients with ≥3 unformed stools, in 24 hours, that are both unexplained and new-onset are the preferred target population for CDI testing. Other factors that contribute to the decision to test include likelihood of infection, risk factors for CDI, available testing methods, and potential confounders (eg, underlying disease, laxative or other medication use) (rules out options B, C, and D). Health care providers can improve testing results by testing only those with diarrhea that cannot be explained by another cause. Laboratories can improve testing by rejecting stool specimens that are not liquid or soft, and by collaborating with quality improvement teams to ensure the appropriate patient population is being tested.[1]

4. **Explanation:** The correct answer is D. The best testing recommendation is based on whether the institution has preagreed criteria for submission of patient stool samples (commonly submitted stool samples versus stool samples from patients likely to have CDI based on clinical symptoms). There are several testing methods that can aid in a diagnosis of CDI and vary in their sensitivity and specificity. Additionally, testing methods and protocols are institution specific and based on laboratory capabilities, costs, and other factors. Options include those that detect the organism or one of its toxins (option A or B) in the stool. Stool toxin enzyme immunoassays (EIAs), once a mainstay of therapy, have variable performance, high costs, take a long time for completion, and have been replaced by newer methods with greater reliability. Stool toxin tests still have utility in testing algorithms, but are no longer used alone. Glutamate dehydrogenase (GDH) enzyme immunoassay detects a common antigen in all isolates of *C. difficile*, but must be combined with a toxin test since it doesn't discriminate against toxigenic and nontoxigenic strains. Nucleic acid amplification tests (NAAT), such as polymerase chain reaction (PCR), are more sensitive than toxin EIAs and GDH. Based on data, PCR is the most reliable diagnostic method when applied to patients who meet the clinical criteria for CDI testing (with ≥ 3 unformed stools, in 24 hours, that are both unexplained and new-onset). This test is quick to perform, and is becoming the test of choice. Therefore, in patients meeting clinical criteria, and when there are preagreed institutional criteria for patient stool submission, the use of NAAT alone or a multistep algorithm (ie, GDH + toxin; GDH + toxin, arbitrated by NAAT; or NAAT + toxin) is preferred. If there are no preagreed criteria, a stool toxin test should be employed as part of a multistep algorithm rather than NAAT alone.[1]

5. **Explanation:** The correct answer is A. Current guidelines recommend oral vancomycin or fidaxomicin as the mainstay of therapy for CDI. Oral administration is preferred due to negligible absorption and the potential for few systemic adverse effects. Metronidazole, which still

has a role in therapy, has fallen out of favor as a first-line agent due to inferior clinical response rates compared to vancomycin (rules out option B). Additionally, repeated or prolonged courses of metronidazole pose the risk of cumulative and irreversible neurotoxicity; therefore, metronidazole use should be limited. CDI cases are classified as initial (new episode of symptoms and positive assay with no symptoms and positive assay within the previous 8 weeks) or recurrent (episode with positive symptoms and diagnostic assay following a confirmed episode within the previous 2 to 8 weeks). Furthermore, initial episodes are stratified as non-severe, severe, or fulminant based on clinical findings. Leukocytosis >15,000 cells/mL or a serum creatinine of >1.5 mg/dL are the accepted criteria used to define severe CDI. Fulminant cases are defined by hypotension, shock, ileus, or megacolon. These criteria are based on expert opinion rather than firm evidence and may require revision as more evidence is obtained. Treatment selection is based on this classification and stratification. Because AH's CDI is classified as an initial episode, and is severe based on his clinical parameters (WBC = 18.1×10^3 mm^3; serum creatinine = 1.7 mg/dL), options C and D can be ruled out. Other treatment strategies include discontinuing therapy with antibiotic agents, if possible, and starting empiric antibiotics in situations where diagnosis may be delayed.[1]

6. **Explanation:** The correct answer is A. Repeat testing (within 7 days) during the same episode of diarrhea is not recommended unless there are significant changes in the patient's clinical presentation due to false-positive results, unnecessary retesting, and low diagnostic yields. In the setting of recurrent CDI, repeat testing is warranted via a toxin test. Retesting to establish cure is discouraged as many patients will remain *C. difficile* positive after successful treatment. Therefore, the most appropriate monitoring and follow-up is to evaluate for resolution of diarrhea and other signs and symptoms of ongoing infection.[1]

7. **Explanation:** The correct answers are A, B, and E. *C. difficile* transmission, in the health care setting, occurs as a result of person-to-person contact (via the fecal-oral route) on the contaminated hands of health care providers. As such, health care providers must use gloves, gowns, and appropriate hand hygiene when caring for this patient population. Hand hygiene should be performed before and after the care of patients with CDI and after glove removal. The methods for hand hygiene include washing with either soap and water or an alcohol-based hand rub. However, hand hygiene with soap and water is preferred over alcohol-based products given superior spore removal with soap and water (*C. difficile* spores are highly resistant to killing with alcohol), especially during outbreaks or if there is direct contact with feces or an area where fecal contamination may have occurred (rules out option C). Environmental contamination is also thought to contribute to the spread of CDI, and precautions should be taken to

safeguard against environmental spread of disease, including: isolation, dedicated/disposable patient care equipment, and appropriate environmental cleaning. Isolation of CDI patients is recommended in patients with suspected or confirmed CDI, and for 48 hours following resolution of diarrhea. At this time, there is no evidence to support contact precautions in asymptomatic carriers (rules out option D). Finally, antibiotic stewardship has good evidence and may be one of the most helpful methods for controlling rates of CDI. Limiting the frequency and duration of antibiotics (especially high-risk antibiotics)

at the patient and ward-level is critical to helping control outbreaks of CDI.[1]

REFERENCE

1. McDonald LC, Gerding DN, Johnson S, et al. Clinical practice guidelines for *Clostridium difficile* infection in adults and children: 2017 update by the Infectious Diseases Society of America (IDSA) and Society for Healthcare Epidemiology of America (SHEA). *Clin Infect Dis.* 2018;66:e1-e48.

23 Traveler's Diarrhea

Amber B. Giles

PATIENT PRESENTATION

Chief Complaint

"I can't stop going to the bathroom, and I'm starting to get dehydrated."

History of Present Illness

JB is a 32-year-old Caucasian male who presents to his primary care physician with complaints of bloody diarrhea approximately 5 times per day, abdominal pain, and nausea for the past 4 days. He also complains of intermittent fevers and dry mouth. He states that he recently traveled to India on a medical mission trip with other students in his medical school program. Of note, JB did not receive any vaccinations or medications prior to travel and has not received antibiotics in the past 5 years. He is up-to-date on all routine childhood vaccines.

Past Medical History

Seasonal allergies, depression, anxiety

Surgical History

Tonsillectomy and adenoidectomy in primary school

Family History

Father has hyperlipidemia and type 2 diabetes; mother has no significant medical history

Social History

Student in his third year of medical school, married, lives with wife, and drinks alcohol occasionally. Reports no illicit drug or tobacco use

Allergies

Ciprofloxacin (hives/shortness of breath)

Home Medications

Cetirizine 10 mg PO daily
Sertraline 100 mg PO daily

Physical Examination

▶ **Vital Signs**

Temp 102.3°F, P 89, RR 24 breaths per minute, BP 110/69 mm Hg, pO$_2$ 94%, Ht 6'2", Wt 89 kg

▶ **General**

Male with dizziness and in mild distress

▶ **HEENT**

Normocephalic, PERRLA, EOMI, dry mucous membranes and conjunctiva, fair dentition

▶ **Pulmonary**

Normal breath sounds

▶ **Cardiovascular**

NSR, no m/r/g

▶ **Abdomen**

Slightly distended, positive for abdominal pain, bowel sounds hyperactive

▶ **Genitourinary**

Normal male genitalia, no complaints of dysuria or hematuria

▶ **Neurology**

Oriented to place and person

▶ **Extremities**

Negative for pain or rash

▶ **Back**

Negative for back pain

Laboratory Findings

Na = 148 mEq/L	K = 3.0 mEq/L	Cl = 107 mEq/L
CO$_2$ = 24 mEq/L	BUN = 32 mg/dL	SCr = 1.5 mg/dL
Glu = 90 mg/dL	Ca = 8.4 mg/dL	Mg = 1.5 mg/dL
Phos = 4.8 mg/dL	Hgb = 15.0 g/dL	Hct = 50%
Plt = 200 × 10^3/mm^3	WBC = 15 × 10^3 mm^3	AST = 18 IU/L
ALT = 20 IU/L	T Bili = 1.4 mg/dL	Alk Phos = 62 IU/L

▶ **Stool Cultures**

Pending

QUESTIONS

1. Which of the following organisms are most likely to cause bloody diarrhea and fever in an international traveler such as JB?
   A. Norovirus
   B. *Clostridioides difficile*
   C. *Salmonella enterica*
   D. All of the above

2. What is the most appropriate management of JB's moderate dehydration?
   A. Oral intake of fluids such as Gatorade or apple juice
   B. Oral rehydration solution (ORS)
   C. Intravenous normal saline
   D. No intervention is needed at this point

3. Which empiric antibiotic regimen would you recommend for JB?
   A. Azithromycin 1,000 mg PO daily for one dose
   B. Ciprofloxacin 500 mg PO daily for one dose
   C. Amoxicillin-clavulanate 875-125 mg PO q12h for one day
   D. Empiric antibiotic therapy is not appropriate in this patient

4. JB is concerned about his wife being exposed to his infection. He asks if she needs to be prescribed an antibiotic as well for empiric treatment. He states that she currently has no signs of infection and has no known drug allergies. What is the most appropriate response to this inquiry?
   A. Recommend an additional dose of azithromycin 1,000 mg for JB's wife
   B. Recommend ciprofloxacin 500 mg PO once
   C. Recommend appropriate infection prevention measures, such as regular hand hygiene
   D. Recommend both B & C

5. Based on JB's presentation, what should be recommended in regard to adjunctive antidiarrheal medications?
   A. Initiate loperamide 4 mg PO once, followed by 2 mg PO after each subsequent stool
   B. Initiate diphenoxylate-atropine 5 mg-0.05 mg 4 times daily
   C. Initiate bismuth subsalicylate 525 mg PO 4 times daily
   D. Antidiarrheal medications are inappropriate in this patient

6. Which of the following preventative measures should be taken to prevent traveler's diarrhea in a patient traveling to a resource-limited country?
   A. Avoid eating raw or undercooked foods, including seafood and meats
   B. Avoid drinking tap water (including ice)
   C. Wash hands frequently using soap and water or hand sanitizer, if needed
   D. All of the above

7. Which of the following is true in regard to prophylaxis against typhoid fever?
   A. Typhim Vi is a live attenuated oral vaccine that should be given prior to travel in areas of moderate to high risk for exposure
   B. Vivotif is an inactivated oral vaccine that should be given prior to travel in areas of moderate to high risk for exposure
   C. Either vaccine will be >90% effective in preventing typhoid fever
   D. Food and hand-washing precautions are recommended in addition to either of the available vaccines

ANSWERS

1. **Explanation:** The correct answer is C. Norovirus typically presents as a watery diarrhea. Additionally, *C. difficile* does not usually present as a bloody diarrhea, and JB has not been exposed to antimicrobials in the recent past. Common causes of bloody diarrhea and fever in immunocompetent patients who have recently travelled include *Salmonella enterica*, *Shigella*, and *Campylobacter* spp.[1]

2. **Explanation:** The correct answer is B. Current guidelines and the CDC recommend ORS as first-line management of mild to moderate dehydration caused by diarrhea.[1,2] If JB is unable to tolerate oral intake, ORS may be administered via nasogastric routes as well.[1] Beverages with high sugar content, such as apple juice, may actually cause osmotic diarrhea if consumed in large quantities. Intravenous solutions such as normal saline and lactated ringer's should be reserved for severe cases of dehydration, altered mental status, and/or shock or in cases where ORS has failed. Once rehydration has been achieved, ongoing losses should be replaced with ORS until the diarrhea has resolved.[1]

3. **Explanation:** The correct answer is A. Current guidelines and the CDC recommend empiric antibiotic therapy in an immunocompetent adult with bloody diarrhea plus a temperature >101.3°F and/or signs of sepsis who have travelled internationally recently.[1,2] JB's recorded temperature is 102.3°F and recently travelled to India. Azithromycin or fluoroquinolone antibiotics are recommended empirically in cases of travelers' diarrhea;[1] however, JB is allergic to ciprofloxacin (hives and shortness of breath). Additionally, azithromycin is the preferred treatment for inflammatory diarrhea due to increasing ciprofloxacin resistance.[2] Taking into account all of this information, azithromycin would be the most appropriate agent for this patient.

4. **Explanation:** The correct answer is C. Current guidelines state that contacts of patients with infectious diarrhea should not be prescribed empiric antibiotics if contacts are currently asymptomatic[1]; therefore, answers A and B are incorrect. Appropriate infection control measures should

be followed, such as contact precautions and appropriate hand hygiene. To prevent transmission of the infectious agent, infected persons should refrain from preparing food or working in childcare settings during periods of diarrheal illness.[1]

5. **Explanation:** The correct answer is D. Adults with bloody diarrhea and fever are not candidates for antimotility therapy.[1] Slowing of fecal transit time may worsen symptoms or lead to gastrointestinal damage and complications in patients with bloody, inflammatory diarrhea. In cases of acute watery diarrhea in immunocompetent adult patients, antimotility agents may be considered to reduce the number of stools; however, it is important to note that these medications should never be used as a substitute for fluid and electrolyte therapies.[1]

6. **Explanation:** The correct answer is D. "Boil it, cook it, peel it, or forget it" is a common saying in regard to preparing foods in resource-limited countries.[2] All meat should be cooked well, and fruits and vegetables should be peeled or cooked by the traveler. Any raw fruits or vegetables that cannot be peeled should not be consumed. Additionally, it is important for travelers to avoid drinking tap water, ice, beverages prepared with tap water such as tea or reconstituted fruit juice, or unpasteurized milk and dairy products. Good personal hygiene should be practiced in order to prevent travel-related illnesses as well. Hand washing with soap and water or alcohol-based sanitizers should be used regularly, which is extremely important before handling or preparing foods.[2]

7. **Explanation:** The correct answer is D. Two vaccines are indeed available for protection against typhoid fever in patients traveling to moderate- to high-risk international destinations.[3] Typhim Vi is an inactivated intramuscular injection that should be given once at least 2 weeks prior to travel, and a booster should be administered every 2 years in patients at continued risk. Vivotif is a live attenuated oral vaccine that should be given every other day for 4 doses and completed at least 1 week prior to travel. This vaccine should be boosted every 5 years in those at continued risk. Each of the vaccines are only 50–80% effective in preventing typhoid fever, so food and hand-washing precautions are still of utmost importance when traveling.[3]

REFERENCES

1. Shane AL, Mody RK, Crump JA, et al. 2017 Infectious Diseases Society of America clinical practice guidelines for the diagnosis and management of infectious diarrhea. *Clin Infect Dis.* 2017;65(12):1963-1973.

2. Connor BA. Travelers' diarrhea: CDC health information for international travel. Centers for Disease Control and Prevention; 2017. Available at https://wwwnc.cdc.gov/travel/yellowbook/2018/the-pre-travel-consultation/travelers-diarrhea. New York, NY, 2018.

3. Judd MC, Mintz ED. Typhoid & paratyphoid fever: CDC Health Information for International Travel. Centers for Disease Control and Prevention; 2017. Available at https://wwwnc.cdc.gov/travel/yellowbook/2018/infectious-diseases-related-to-travel/typhoid-paratyphoid-fever. New York, NY, 2018.

24 Hepatitis C

Lindsey Childs-Kean

PATIENT PRESENTATION

Chief Complaint

"I want to get this Hepatitis C cured."

History of Present Illness

PD is a 45-year-old Caucasian male who presents to the infectious diseases clinic seeking treatment for his chronic hepatitis C infection. He states that he was diagnosed with the disease a few years ago, but he's not sure when he contracted it. He doesn't remember having any symptoms related to the infection. He has never received any treatment for his hepatitis C.

Past Medical History

HTN, anxiety, dyslipidemia, GERD

Surgical History

None

Family History

Father and mother both alive with HTN and dyslipidemia; sister is alive with no known medical issues.

Social History

Former IV drug user and alcohol drinker, but clean and sober for 7+ years. No tobacco. Works repairing wheelchairs and scooters. Married with 2 children (12 and 4 years). Enjoys playing sports and doing outdoor activities with wife and children.

Allergies

NKDA

Home Medications

Amlodipine 10 mg PO daily
Alprazolam 1 mg PO TID PRN for anxiety
Simvastatin 20 mg PO daily
Omeprazole 40 mg PO daily
Multivitamin PO daily
Acetaminophen 325 mg PO PRN for headache

Physical Examination

▸ **Vital Signs**

Temp 98.8°F, P 82 bpm, RR 18 breaths per minute, BP 127/78 mm Hg, pO_2 99%, Ht 6′, Wt 101 kg

▸ **General**

Normal appearing male in no apparent distress, well groomed

▸ **HEENT**

Nomocephalic, atraumatic, PERRLA, EOMI, b/l sclera anicteric, moist mucous membranes, poor dentition

▸ **Pulmonary**

Clear to auscultation, no use of accessory muscles, no cracks or wheezes

▸ **Cardiovascular**

NSR, no m/r/g

▸ **Abdomen**

Soft, non-distended, non-tender, normal bowel sounds

▸ **Genitourinary**

Normal male genitalia, no complaints of dysuria or hematuria

▸ **Neurology**

Alert and oriented × 3, CN 2-12 grossly intact

▸ **Extremities**

No edema, cyanosis, or clubbing

▸ **Skin**

Intact, w/o rashes or lesions, or erythema

Laboratory Findings

WBC: 6×10^9 cells/L	Glucose: 80 mg/dL	Albumin: 3.8 mg/dL
Hgb: 15 g/dL	BUN: 15 mg/dL	T bili: 0.8 mg/dL
Hct: 45%	SCr: 0.9 mg/dL	AST/ALT: 50 IU/L / 50 IU/L
Plts: 102,000/mmol	K: 4 mEq/L	Alk Phos: 100 IU/L

Hgb A1C: 5%   Na: 140 mEq/L   Total Chol: 180 mg/dL

TSH: 2 mIU/L CO_2: 22 mEq/L   HDL: 65 mg/dL

INR: 1.3   Ca: 8.5 mg/dL   LDL: 90 mg/dL

Cl: 100 mEq/L   Triglycerides: 150 mg/dL

Hepatitis C Genotype = 1a
Hepatitis C Viral Load = 8,237,625 IU/mL
Hepatitis A Antibody Total = Negative
Hepatitis B sAg Screen = Negative
Hepatitis B cAb Total = Negative
Hepatitis B sAb = Negative
Liver biopsy (2016) = Cirrhosis, inflammation grade 3 out of 4
Resistance-Associated Substitutions = None detected

QUESTIONS

1. What is the most likely route from which PD contracted hepatitis C?
   A. Alcohol use
   B. Sexual activity
   C. IV drug use
   D. Eating contaminated food

2. What is this patient's Child–Pugh score? Correspondingly, how would PD's degree of liver fibrosis/cirrhosis be staged?
   A. Score: 0, No fibrosis
   B. Score: 5, Bridging fibrosis
   C. Score: 5, Compensated cirrhosis
   D. Score: 8, Decompensated cirrhosis

3. At what time point does the viral load need to be undetectable in order for the patient to achieve a sustained virological response, the goal of treatment, which is regarded as a "virological cure"?
   A. At the end of treatment
   B. 4 weeks after treatment ends
   C. 8 weeks after treatment ends
   D. 12 weeks after treatment ends

4. Which of the patient's current medications does NOT cause any drug–drug interactions with the four recommended hepatitis C regimens for treatment naïve genotype 1a patients[1] (sofosbuvir/ledipasvir, sofosbuvir/velpatasvir, glecaprevir/pibrentasvir, and elbasvir/grazoprevir)?
   A. Amlodipine
   B. Alprazolam
   C. Simvastatin
   D. Omeprazole

5. Which regimen would you recommend for the treatment of PD's chronic hepatitis C without having to change any of his other medications?
   A. Elbasvir/grazoprevir
   B. Glecaprevir/pibrentasvir
   C. Sofosbuvir/ledipasvir
   D. Sofosbuvir/velpatasvir

6. What is the recommended duration of treatment if PD is to be treated with elbasvir/grazoprevir?
   A. 12 weeks
   B. 16 weeks
   C. 24 weeks
   D. Not enough information to answer

7. In addition to the hepatitis C viral load, what laboratory findings should be monitored as PD undergoes treatment for his hepatitis C? (limit to laboratory findings relevant to hepatitis C disease and antiviral treatment)
   A. Serum creatinine, albumin, total bilirubin, AST/ALT, alkaline phosphatase
   B. CBC, serum creatinine, AST/ALT
   C. CBC, serum creatinine, albumin, total bilirubin, AST/ALT, alkaline phosphatase
   D. CBC, TSH, albumin, total bilirubin

8. Based on PD's hepatitis A and B serologies, what, if any, hepatitis vaccinations does he need to receive?
   A. No vaccinations needed
   B. Hepatitis A only
   C. Hepatitis B only
   D. Hepatitis A and B

ANSWERS

1. **Explanation:** The correct answer is C. Hepatitis C is most commonly transmitted by blood to blood contact. Since the blood supply has been able to be screened (mid-1990s), the most common route of transmission is IV drug use. Since the patient has a history of IV drug use, this is likely the way he was infected with hepatitis C. Hepatitis C can be transmitted sexually, but it is very rare in heterosexual monogamous couples. Alcohol use and eating contaminated food are not routes of transmission of hepatitis C.

2. **Explanation:** The correct answer is C. The patient's liver biopsy shows cirrhosis, which is stage 4 of 4 fibrosis (Stage 1 is no fibrosis and Stage 3 is bridging fibrosis). According to Child–Pugh, which looks at INR, total bilirubin, albumin, presence or absence of ascites, and presence or absence of hepatic encephalopathy, the patient has compensated cirrhosis with a Child–Pugh score of 5.

3. **Explanation:** The correct answer is D. Sustained virological response is defined as an undetectable viral load at least 12 weeks following the end of treatment for chronic hepatitis C.

4. **Explanation:** The correct answer is B. Simvastatin is a substrate of the OATP1B1/3, BCRP, and P-gp transporters, so the plasma levels of simvastatin are going to increase significantly with an inhibitor of those transporters, like glecaprevir/pibrentasvir, sofosbuvir/ledipasvir, and sofosbuvir/velpatasvir. Amlodipine is a substrate of the P-gp transporter, and ledipasvir is an inhibitor of that transporter. Omeprazole reduces the acidity of the stomach,

and absorption of ledipasvir and velpatasvir is significantly reduced with less acidity in the stomach. Alprazolam is the only drug listed free of drug–drug interactions with the common hepatitis C regimens.

5. **Explanation:** The correct answer is A. Glecaprevir/pibrentasvir is contraindicated with simvastatin use. PD's current dose of omeprazole is above the recommended max dose (20 mg) that is to be given concurrently with ledipasvir or velpatasvir. Elbasvir/grazoprevir does potentially interact with simvastatin, but only monitoring of side effects is recommended.

6. **Explanation:** The correct answer is A. Patients who have genotype 1a (as PD does) and are going to receive elbasvir/grazoprevir need to have baseline resistance testing done, looking for resistance-associated substitutions (RASs) to the NS5A inhibitor (elbasvir in this case). Since PD has no RASs, then the patient should receive 12 weeks of treatment. If he had had at least one RAS, then the patient should have received 16 weeks of treatment.

7. **Explanation:** The correct answer is A. A complete blood count (CBC) is only recommended if a patient is receiving ribavirin as a part of treatment due to its risk of anemia. PD is not receiving ribavirin, so a CBC does not need to be monitored. Serum creatinine and a hepatic function panel (including albumin, total bilirubin, AST/ALT, alkaline phosphatase) are recommended at 4 weeks into treatment and then as indicated.

8. **Explanation:** The correct answer is D. PD has a negative hepatitis A antibody, so he needs to receive the hepatitis A vaccination series. He is also negative for both the hepatitis B core and surface antibodies, so he needs the hepatitis B vaccination series as well.

REFERENCE

1. AASLD-IDSA. Recommendations for testing, managing, and treating hepatitis C. Available at http://www.hcvguidelines.org. 2019.

25 Syphilis

Trent G. Towne

PATIENT PRESENTATION

Chief Complaint

"I think I am allergic to something."

History of Present Illness

JS is a 27-year-old man who presents to a free health clinic at the county hospital. He states he was in his usual state of health until about 3 days ago when he began developing a rash on his stomach that is now on the palms of his hands and soles of his feet. The rash is not painful or itchy. He states that he had this strange little "ulcer-like" thing on his penis a couple weeks ago but it went away and never really hurt. He is single and sexually active with two to three concurrent male partners. He has had unprotected sex with "at least one of his partners" in the past couple of weeks. He doesn't know the sexual histories of his current or past sexual partners, and admits to over 15 lifetime partners. He endorses rectal and oral sex. He doesn't ever recall being tested for HIV, and knows he received all his childhood vaccines, "cause my mom told me." He has never been vaccinated against HPV stating, "that's a woman's disease," and is unsure if he ever has received a hepatitis A vaccine.

Past Medical History

None

Surgical History

None

Family History

Father had HTN and passed away from a stroke 4 years ago; mother is still living and has type 2 DM

Social History

MSM with multiple sexual partners; (+) EtOH, (–) Tobacco, (+) Marijuana, (–) Illicit drugs

Allergies

NKDA

Home Medications

Ibuprofen 200 mg PO PRN pain (has taken 4 doses in the last day)

Physical Examination

▶ **Vital Signs**

Temp 101°F, P 72, RR 16 breaths per minute, BP 141/85 mm Hg, pO$_2$ 94%, Ht 5'7", Wt 60 kg

▶ **General**

NAD, awake, alert, slightly underweight man

▶ **Skin**

Diffuse mucocutaneous rash noted on abdomen, back, upper extremities (including palms of hands) and soles of feet; macules are easy to blanch and are not associated with any area of fluctuance

▶ **HEENT**

PERRLA; EOMI; mucous membranes are moist and neck is supple without any evidence of lymphadenopathy

▶ **Pulmonary**

Clear auscultation with no wheezing or rhonci

▶ **Cardiovascular**

NSR; no m/r/g

▶ **Abdomen**

NTND with no rebounding or guarding; (+) BS; noted rash as described above

▶ **Genitourinary**

Abdominal rash extends to genital region and base of penis; noted healing wound/ulcer on the dorsal aspect of the penis

▶ **Neurology**

CN II-XII intact

▶ **Extremities**

Well-perfused and warm to the touch; noted rash as described above

Laboratory Findings

Na =136 mEq/L	Hgb = 11.4 g/dL
K = 4.1 mEq/L	Hct = 35%
Cl = 98 mEq/L	Plt = 141 × 10^3/mm³
CO_2 = 26 mEq/L	WBC = 10.2 × 10^3 mm³
BUN = 14 mg/dL	AST = 54 IU/L
SCr = 0.96 mg/dL	ALT = 85 IU/L
Glu = 101 mg/dL	T. Bili = 4.9 mg/dL

▶ *Additional Testing*

RPR: Positive with a titer of 1:128
TP-EIA: Positive
CSF-VDRL: Non-reactive
Hepatitis A: HAV IgM Ab: Negative
Hepatitis B: HBsAb: Positive; HBsAg: Negative
Hepatitis C: RNA negative

QUESTIONS

1. Which pathogen is most likely causing this patient's current symptoms?
   A. *Mycoplasma genitalium*
   B. *Chlamydia trachomatis*
   C. *Treponema pallidum*
   D. *Staphylococcus aureus*

2. Which additional testing could be done to confirm JS's diagnosis of syphilis?
   A. Darkfield microscopy
   B. Acid-fast bacilli staining
   C. KOH testing
   D. Gram staining

3. What is the clinical stage of JS's syphilis?
   A. Primary
   B. Secondary
   C. Tertiary
   D. Neurosyphilis

4. What would be the most appropriate therapeutic choice for JS's syphilis?
   A. Benzathine Penicillin G 2.4 million units IM × 1 dose
   B. Benzathine Penicillin G 2.4 million units IM × 3 doses separated by one week
   C. Aqueous Penicillin G 20 million units IV continuous infusion daily for 10 days
   D. Aqueous Penicillin G 24 million units IM daily × 3 doses

5. One day after starting therapy for syphilis, JS begins to experience fever, muscle pain, and headache. What is the most likely explanation for these findings?
   A. Allergic reaction
   B. Stevens–Johnson syndrome
   C. Jarisch–Herxheimer reaction
   D. Treatment failure

6. After completing the correct treatment for his syphilis, what is the most appropriate recommendation for follow-up of his infection?
   A. No further follow-up is required
   B. He should have a follow-up RPR test at 6 months
   C. He should have a follow-up FTA-ABS test at 12 months
   D. He should return to a primary care provider for evaluation of his clinical response in 1 week

7. What additional screening should be performed for JS because of his diagnosis of syphilis?
   A. HIV
   B. Urine drug screen
   C. HPV
   D. Tuberculosis

8. If JS had presented with a type-1 allergy to penicillin, what would be the most appropriate antibiotic regimen to consider for his therapy
   A. Doxycycline 100 mg PO BID × 10 days
   B. Ceftriaxone 1g IV daily × 14 days
   C. Levofloxacin 750 mg PO daily × 10 days
   D. Rifampin 300 mg PO TID × 14 days

ANSWERS

1. **Explanation:** The correct answer is C. *Treponema pallidum* is the causative pathogen for the sexually transmitted infection, syphilis. In this case, JS has several symptoms that point toward a diagnosis of syphilis including the mucocutaneous rash on the abdomen, fever, and prior history of the ulcer on his penis. Additionally, he has one of the most common risk factors for syphilis, being a man who has sex with men (MSM). This correlates with the positive RPR and TP-EIA results, two tests used in the diagnosis of syphilis. Serologic testing is the mainstay of diagnostic testing for syphilis and comes in two different antibody tests, nontreponemal and treponemal tests. Rapid plasma reagin test (RPR) is the primary nontreponemal test that can be used in screening for syphilis and can serve as a marker to gauge response to treatment. Another nontreponemal test that is utilized in practice is the Venereal Disease Research Laboratory (VDRL) test. While still a quantitative assay, VDRL results cannot be compared to the RPR, as RPR titers are usually higher than VDRL. VDRL testing has been largely replaced by RPR for general screening of patients with suspected syphilis, but it still is widely used to evaluate CNS disease. Several treponemal tests are also available for making the diagnosis of syphilis. The role of treponemal testing as either a screening tool or conformation test is still evolving in modern practice. Nontreponemal tests include fluorescent treponemal antibody absorbed test (FTA-ABS), microhemagglutination test for antibodies to *T. pallidum* (MHA-TP), *T. pallidum* particle agglutination assay (TP-PA), *T. pallidum* enzyme assay (TP-EIA), and chemiluminescence immunoassay (CIA). The conventional treponemal tests (FTA-ABS and

MHA-TP) have been largely replaced by TP-PA, EIA, and CIA testing due to ease of use and automated technologies. Regardless, the results for treponemal testing will remain positive for life, even with effective treatment.[1,2] Answer choices A and B both represent pathogens capable of causing STIs; however, JS's symptoms do not correlate with the presentation of those organisms. Additionally, answer choice D would be incorrect because *S. aureus* is usually associated with fluctuant skin and soft tissue infections rather than generalized cellulitis.

2. **Explanation:** The correct answer is A. Direct detection of *T. pallidum* is another methodology that can be used in the diagnosis of syphilis, however for many reasons serologic testing is preferred. Examples of direct methods of detection of syphilis include darkfield microscopy, direct fluorescent antibody test for *T. pallidum* (DFA-TP), silver staining, and PCR testing. Darkfield microscopy is a rapid, direct method of confirming the presence of *T. pallidum*. Its use is limited by the need to investigate only motile treponomes, which requires special equipment and highly trained personnel to utilize. Much like darkfield microscopy, direct fluorescent antibody test for *T. pallidum* (DFA-TP) also requires highly specialized equipment and is technically complex to conduct. Silver staining of *T. pallidum* in tissue fixed with formalin also represents a traditional method for direct detection; however, it lacks specificity for only *T. pallidum* and has limited sensitivity. PCR testing represents the final example of direct detection of *T. pallidum*, and while PCR has been successfully employed in a number of infectious disease diagnostic tools, in the setting of syphilis there is no commercially available testing. In addition, this method will amplify the DNA of living and dead bacteria, leading to the potential for false-positive results. Answer choice B would be correct only for mycobacterial species (*T. pallidum* is a spirochete). Answer choice C would be correct for a number of STI-associated vaginal discharge, but since JS is a man this would not be an incorrect answer. Answer D is not correct because although a bacterium *T. pallidum* does not stain by traditional bacterial Gram-staining methods.[1,2]

3. **Explanation:** The correct answer is B. This patient has secondary syphilis as is evidenced by the systemic nature of his symptoms including the mucocutaneous rash on his abdomen, palms of his hands and soles of his feet, and his fever. While secondary syphilis can impact all organ systems, over 95% of patients will experience lesions of the skin and mucous membranes. Patients with primary syphilis will present with an ulcer, or chancre, that is usually painless, has a raised border, and is without exudate. JW did identify a healed, non-painful ulcer on his penis that resolved 2 weeks ago, making it likely that was the primary stage of syphilis (eliminating answer choice A). The absence of pain from the chancre is also helpful in the differentiation of primary syphilis from other STIs such as *Haemophilus ducreyi* and herpes simplex virus which

also can cause genital ulceration. Left untreated, primary syphilis would progress to the symptoms JS is currently observing as secondary syphilis. At either the primary or secondary state of syphilis a patient may develop neurosyphilis. While many patients will remain asymptomatic and even resolve their neurosyphilis, those who do develop disease may exhibit a wide array of syndromes including meningitis, meningovascular disease, cranial neuritis, and occular disease that may overlap. JW's treponemal serum titers are positive, but his CSF-VDRL is negative and he is exhibiting no signs or symptoms of meningitis (eliminating answer choice D). Patients who are not treated, or who are undertreated, in the secondary phase of syphilis may also simply resolve their signs and symptoms of infection progress to latent syphilis. Latent syphilis can be further subdivided into early latent (<1 year from infection) and late latent (>1 year from infection) types. During early latent syphilis, relapses of infection with or without spirochetemia are common; however, in late latent syphilis these relapses and bloodstream infections are uncommon. Tertiary syphilis usually produces illness >5 years after the initial infection (eliminating answer choice C). Much like the other stages of syphilis, tertiary syphilis can be subdivided into cardiovascular, gummatous, and some forms of neurosyphilis.[1,2]

4. **Explanation:** The correct answer is A. Penicillin G is the correct antibiotic choice for this patient; however, route of administration, dose, and duration are the defining features for this answer as syphilis treatment is based on stage of disease. For patients with primary, secondary, or early latent syphilis, a single dose of benzathine penicillin G 2.4 million units, given as a one-time dose intramuscularly, is the most appropriate therapy. It should be noted that Bicillin L-A (standard benzathine penicillin G) and Bicillin C-R (benzathine-procaine penicillin G) are not interchangeable. Only Bicillin L-A should be utilized in the management of primary, secondary, or early latent syphilis as using Bicillin C-R may result in not fully treating the patient. Answer choice B, while correct in dose and route, is incorrect with regard to the duration of therapy of 3 weeks. This duration would be more consistent with the diagnosis of tertiary or late, latent syphilis. Aqueous penicillin G given as IM or IV is recommended only for the treatment of neurosyphilis (eliminating answer choices C and D).[1]

5. **Explanation:** The correct answer is C. This patient is experiencing a Jarisch–Herxheimer reaction which can occur with the initiation of treatment for syphilis at any stage of the disease, but most commonly in the primary and secondary phases. It most commonly occurs within 6 to 8 hours of the initiation of treatment and lasts for 12 to 24 hours. The reaction is thought to be due to a cytokine storm in response to the lysing and death of the trepononemes. While it can vary in severity, symptom onset is usually abrupt and can include fever, chills, headache,

myalgias, mild hypotension, vasodilation with flushing, hyperventilation, and tachycardia. Broadly speaking, symptoms can be managed by anti-inflammatory agents and/or antipyretics. Though commonly confused with an allergic reaction (especially in patients with secondary syphilis who have a rash), it is not an allergic reaction (eliminating answer choice A). Stevens–Johnson syndrome can occur as a result of drug therapy; however, this does not usually occur until 1 to 3 weeks after the initiation of therapy, and is usually associated with skin blisters that easily slough off (eliminating answer choice B). Since the patient has only been on therapy for one day, failure of therapy cannot be assessed at this point (eliminating answer choice D).[1,2]

6. **Explanation:** The correct answer is B. The patient should have serology, with non-treponemal testing (eg, RPR), completed at 6 and 12 months. Treponemal testing would not provide any additional information as the patient will likely have a positive result for the rest of his life and treatment will not result in any decline in the positivity of this result (eliminating answer choice C). Evaluation of the clinical response is not necessary until the 6-month mark unless the patient has not observed a significant resolution in the signs and symptoms of his infection (eliminating answer choices A and D).[1]

7. **Explanation:** The correct answer is A. Patients who are diagnosed with any sexually transmitted infection should be screened for HIV. While he does have a history of drug use (marijuana), simply being diagnosed with syphilis does not merit screening for this (eliminates answer choice B). HPV infection is a widely disseminated STI; however, there are no recommendations for routine screening of this infection in men, regardless of diagnosis of another sexually transmitted infection (eliminates answer choice C). Tuberculosis, while a common co-infection in patients with HIV, is not directly associated with syphilis; therefore, the screening is not necessary. If the patient is tested for HIV and found to be positive, then tuberculosis screening would be warranted (eliminates answer choice D).[1]

8. **Explanation:** The correct answer is A. In patients with a type 1 penicillin allergy, all beta-lactam antibiotics should be avoided (eliminating answer choice B). This makes the use of a tetracycline antibiotic the preferred agent. While tetracycline would be an okay choice for this patient, using doxycycline for 10 days minimizes the frequency of dosing to promote compliance (ie, BID vs QID) . Neither answer C nor D is routinely used in the management of sexually transmitted infections, including syphilis.[1]

REFERENCES

1. Workowski KA, Bolan GA. Sexually transmitted diseases treatment guidelines 2015. *MMWR Recomm Rep.* 2015; 64(No. RR-3):1-140.
2. Radolf JD, Tramont EC, Salazar JC. Syphilis (*Treponema pallidum*) in principles and practice of infectious disease. 8th ed. In: Bennett JE, Dolin R, Blaser MJ, eds. Philadelphia, PA. Elsevier Saunders; 2015:2684-2709.

26 Herpes

Elias B. Chahine

PATIENT PRESENTATION

Chief Complaint

"I have painful sores in my genital area and I have been feeling achy."

History of Present Illness

JJ is a 20-year-old Caucasian female who presents to the community health center for evaluation of genital lesions that have been present for two days. The lesions are painful, vesicular, and accompanied by inguinal lymphadenopathy. JJ has never experienced these symptoms before. Upon further questioning, she stated that she experienced pain, tingling, itching, and burning sensation before the appearance of the lesions. She admits to having multiple male sex partners within the past six months while she was studying abroad and stated that her last sexual encounter was a week ago. She and her partners occasionally but not always use barrier methods during sexual intercourse. JJ is also complaining of nasal congestion and sneezing.

Past Medical History

Vulvovaginal candidiasis, allergic rhinitis

Surgical History

Appendectomy at age 18

Family History

Father has HTN, mother has T2DM, sister has PCOS

Social History

Lives at home with her parents; enjoys swimming and running; drinks alcohol occasionally; denies tobacco and illicit drug use

Allergies

Penicillin (hives)

Home Medications

Cetirizine 10 mg PO daily
Ethinyl estradiol 0.02 mg and drospirenone 3 mg, one tablet PO daily
Fluticasone furoate (27.5 mcg/spray), one spray in each nostril once daily
Multivitamin, one tablet PO daily

Physical Examination

▶ **Vital Signs**

Temp 100.04°F; BP 118/74 mm Hg; HR 80 beats/minute; RR 18 breaths/minute; Ht 5'6"; Wt 52.3 kg

▶ **General**

Well nourished, mild acute distress

▶ **HEENT**

Normocephalic, atraumatic, PERRLA, EOMI, moist mucus membranes, good dentition

▶ **Cardiovascular**

NSR, no m/r/g

▶ **Abdomen**

Soft, non-distended, non-tender, normal bowel sounds

▶ **Genitourinary**

Small painful unruptured vesicular lesions in the labia majora, redness and inflammation in the surrounding area, tender local inguinal lymphadenopathy

▶ **Neurology**

Alert and oriented ×3

▶ **Extremities**

No edema, no petechiae

Laboratory Findings

Na = 138 mEq/L	Hgb = 15 g/dL	Ca = 8.2 mg/dL
K = 4 mEq/L	Hct = 45%	Mg = 2.3 mg/dL
Cl = 100 mEq/L	Plt = 250 × 10^3/mm³	Phos = 4.6 mg/dL
CO_2 = 28 mEq/L	WBC = 8.2 × 10^3/mm³	AST = 24 IU/L
BUN = 20 mg/dL		ALT = 22 IU/L
SCr = 0.9 mg/dL		T bili = 1.2 mg/dL
Glu = 99 mg/dL		Alk phos = 78 IU/L

▶ **Other Labs**

HSV PCR vaginal swab: (+) for HSV-2; HIV antibodies non-reactive; hCG test negative

QUESTIONS

1. Which of the following is a risk factor for acquiring genital herpes infection?
   A. Drinking alcohol
   B. Having multiple sex partners
   C. Swimming in a community pool
   D. Taking birth control pills

2. What signs and symptoms does JJ have that are consistent with a genital herpes infection?
   A. Fever and nasal congestion
   B. Fever and painful vesicular genital lesions
   C. Nasal congestion and painful vesicular genital lesions
   D. Nasal congestion and sneezing

3. What is the best treatment regimen for JJ's initial episode of genital herpes?
   A. Acyclovir 5 mg/kg IV q8h × 7 days
   B. Acyclovir 400 mg PO TID × 7 days
   C. Famciclovir 125 mg PO BID × 5 days
   D. Valacyclovir 1 g PO daily × 5 days

4. Three months later, JJ calls the community health center complaining of painful lesions in her genital area that look and feel the same as her previous episode from her initial visit. However, there are fewer lesions and they are less painful. What is the best treatment for JJ's lesions at this time?
   A. Acyclovir 400 mg PO TID × 7 days
   B. Famciclovir 250 mg PO TID × 10 days
   C. Valacyclovir 1 g PO daily × 5 days
   D. Valacyclovir 1 g PO BID × 7 days

5. One year later, JJ returns to the community health center complaining of frequent genital herpes recurrences. She is wondering if there is anything that can be done to decrease the frequency of her recurrences. JJ is currently asymptomatic. What is the best recommendation for JJ at this time?
   A. Acyclovir 200 mg PO BID
   B. Famciclovir 250 mg PO daily
   C. Valacyclovir 1 g PO daily
   D. Valacyclovir 500 mg PO BID

6. JJ is now in a relationship with a man she met at recent birthday party. JJ is wondering if there is anything that can be done to prevent transmission of genital herpes to her new boyfriend. What are some important counseling points for the couple to decrease the risk of transmission of genital herpes?
   A. Abstain from sexual intercourse during symptomatic episodes
   B. JJ should continue to take suppressive antiviral therapy
   C. Use condoms consistently and appropriately
   D. All of the above

7. JJ returns to the community health center complaining of a burning, tingling, and itching sensation around her mouth since yesterday. She has had cold sores in the past and was told that she has HSV-1 infection. She is worried about what others will think if she has a breakout of cold sores during graduation and wants to know if there is any medication that she can obtain from the pharmacy without a prescription from the doctor's office. What is the best recommendation for JJ at this time?
   A. Initiate acyclovir 5% cream and apply 5 times daily for 4 days
   B. Initiate acyclovir 5% ointment and apply 6 times daily for 7 days
   C. Initiate docosanol 10% cream at first sign of cold sore and apply 5 times daily until healed
   D. Initiate penciclovir 1% cream at first sign of cold sore and apply every 2 hours while awake for 4 days

ANSWERS

1. **Explanation:** The correct answer is B. Genital herpes is usually acquired through sexual contact with an individual infected with HSV-2. Having multiple sex partners increases the risk for acquiring sexually transmitted diseases including genital herpes. Drinking alcohol, swimming in the community pool, and taking birth control pills do not increase the risk of acquiring genital herpes in the absence of sexual intercourse.[1]

2. **Explanation:** The correct answer is B. Although the clinical manifestation of genital herpes is highly variable, initial presentation may include painful vesicular lesions, tender local inguinal lymphadenopathy, dysuria, fever, and headache. Nasal congestion and sneezing are likely the symptoms of her allergic rhinitis.[1]

3. **Explanation:** The correct answer is B. According to the 2015 CDC guidelines for the treatment of sexually transmitted diseases, acyclovir 400 mg PO TID for 7 to 10 days is one of the recommended regimens for the treatment of the initial episode of genital herpes. Treatment can be extended if healing is incomplete after 10 days of therapy. Intravenous therapy is recommended for patients with severe herpes disease that requires hospitalization such as disseminated infection and CNS manifestations. Famciclovir 125 mg PO BID × 5 days and valacyclovir 1 g PO daily × 5 days are two of the recommended regimens for the episodic treatment of recurrent genital herpes, not initial episodes. All antivirals are considered equally effective and the choice of an agent is influenced by cost, frequency of administration, and duration of therapy. The duration of therapy is usually longer for an initial episode of genital herpes.[1-4]

4. **Explanation:** The correct answer is C. According to the 2015 CDC guidelines for the treatment of sexually transmitted diseases, valacyclovir 1 g PO daily for 5 days is one of the recommended regimens for the episodic treatment of recurrent genital herpes. Acyclovir 400 mg PO TID × 7 days, famciclovir 250 mg PO TID × 10 days, and valacyclovir 1 g PO BID × 7 days are three of the recommended regimens for the treatment of the initial episode of genital

herpes. It is recommended to start treatment as early as possible after symptom onset. All antivirals are considered equally effective and the choice of an agent is influenced by cost, frequency of administration, and duration of therapy. The duration of therapy is usually shorter for a recurrent episode of genital herpes.[1-4]

5. **Explanation:** The correct answer is C. According to the 2015 CDC guidelines for the treatment of sexually transmitted diseases, valacyclovir 1 g PO daily is one of the recommended regimens for the suppressive treatment of recurrent genital herpes. Acyclovir 200 mg PO BID, famciclovir 250 mg PO daily, and valacyclovir 500 mg PO BID are incorrect regimens for the suppressive treatment of recurrent genital herpes. Valacyclovir 500 mg daily is considered less effective than other regimens in patients with 10 or more episodes per year. The choice of an agent is influenced by cost and frequency of administration.[1-4]

6. **Explanation:** The correct answer is D. In order to decrease the risk of transmission of genital herpes, the couple should abstain from sexual intercourse during symptomatic episodes and use condoms consistently and appropriately. Latex condoms or polyurethane condoms in the presence of allergy to latex provide better protection against sexually transmitted diseases than "natural"/lambskin condoms. In addition, JJ should continue to take suppressive antiviral therapy to decrease the risk of genital herpes recurrences. Transmission rates can increase during symptomatic periods. JJ should inform her sexual partners about her infection. Sexual partners should consider testing if they are unaware of their status and should consider receiving treatment if they are infected or if they become symptomatic.[1]

7. **Explanation:** The correct answer is C. Docosanol 10% cream is the only topical antiviral product available over-the-counter for the treatment of herpes labialis. Penciclovir 1% cream and acyclovir 5% cream are used for the treatment of herpes labialis; however, they require a prescription. Acyclovir 5% ointment is used for the treatment of genital herpes and requires a prescription.[5-7]

REFERENCES

1. Centers for Disease Control and Prevention. Sexually transmitted diseases treatment guidelines, 2015. *MMWR.* 2015;64(3):1-137.
2. Zovirax (Acyclovir) [package insert]. Research Triangle Park, NC: GlaxoSmithKline; June 2005.
3. Famvir (Famciclovir). [package insert]. East Hanover, NJ: Novartis Pharmaceuticals Corp; February 2006.
4. Valtrex (Valacyclovir) [package insert]. Research Triangle Park, NC; GlaxoSmithKline; September 2008.
5. Usatine RP, Tinitigan R. Nongenital herpes simplex virus. *Am Fam Physician.* 2010;82:1075-1082.
6. Abreva (Docosanol) [package insert]. Research Triangle Park, NC: GlaxoSmithKline; June 2006.
7. Denavir (Penciclovir) [package insert]. Newtown, PA: Prestium Pharma, Inc; September 2013.

27 Chlamydia and Gonorrhea

Takova D. Wallace-Gay   Jonathan C. Cho

PATIENT PRESENTATION

Chief Complaint

"I've noticed some discharge in my underwear."

History of Present Illness

TP is a 23-year-old black female who presents to the family medicine clinic with complaints of unusual discharge. She reports a frequent sensation of urination and mentions that she has been having odorless vaginal discharge that is different than usual. Upon questioning she mentions being nervous that she may have an STD because she had unprotected vaginal intercourse with a young man after a fraternity party about 2 weeks ago. Since then, she heard rumors that this particular gentleman has a history of multiple sexual partners, but she was not concerned until noticing the discharge 2 days ago.

Past Medical History

Asthma, prior ankle injury

Surgical History

Tonsillectomy

Family History

Mother and father with HTN

Social History

Active as a college basketball player; occasionally smokes marijuana; (–) tobacco; (+) EtOH (beer and liquor most weekends)

Allergies

Doxycycline (swelling of lips and tongue as a teenager)

Home Medications

Acetaminophen 500 mg, two tablets PO q4-6h PRN pain
Ibuprofen 200 mg PO q4-6h PRN pain
Albuterol metered-dose-inhaler 2 puffs q4h PRN shortness of breath and prior to exercise
Ethinyl estradiol and norgestimate (Ortho Tri-Cyclen Lo) one tablet PO daily

Physical Examination

▶ Vital Signs

Temp 98.6°F, P 68, RR 18 breaths per minute, BP 116/70 mm Hg, pO_2 97%, Ht 5'8", Wt 72.7 kg

▶ General

Well developed, well-nourished female in no acute distress

▶ HEENT

Non-contributory

▶ Pulmonary

Denies shortness of breath

▶ Cardiovascular

NSR, no m/r/g

▶ Abdomen

Soft, non-distended, non-tender, (+) bowel sounds

▶ Genitourinary

Normal female genitalia, denies abnormal bleeding, (+) vaginal discharge

▶ Neurology

(+) headaches 1–2 times a week, A&O ×3

▶ Extremities

Noncontributory

Laboratory Findings

Na = 136 mEq/L	Hgb = 12.9 g/dL	Ca = 8.5 mg/dL
K = 4.1 mEq/L	Hct = 37.3%	Mg = 2.1 mEq/L
Cl = 98 mEq/L	Plt = $256 \times 10^3/mm^3$	Phos = 3.5 mg/dL
CO_2 = 26 mEq/L	WBC = $6.3 \times 10^3/mm^3$	AST = 18 U/L
BUN = 12 mg/dL		ALT = 22 U/L
SCr = 0.9 mg/dL		T Bili = 0.2 mg/dL
Glu = 108 mg/dL		Alk Phos = 40 IU/L

Tests Performed

Vaginal discharge: Whiff test (–); yeast (–); wet mount: pending

Urine nucleic acid amplification testing (NAAT): pending

Serology: pending

QUESTIONS

1. Which sexually transmitted infection is TP mostly likely to have?
   A. *Neisseria gonorrhoeae*
   B. *Candida albicans*
   C. *Treponema pallidium*
   D. *Gardnerella vaginalis*

2. Which laboratory test is considered to be the most sensitive and is recommended for detecting *N. gonorrhoeae*?
   A. Wet mount on genital discharge
   B. Serologic (blood antibody) test
   C. Rapid plasma region (RPR) card test
   D. Nucleic acid amplification test (NAAT)

3. If preliminary urine NAAT is positive for *N. gonorrhoeae*, what other sexually transmitted infection should be assumed?
   A. Syphilis
   B. Chlamydia
   C. Genital herpes
   D. Bacterial vaginitis

4. What empiric antimicrobial therapy is most appropriate for TP?
   A. Doxycycline 100 mg PO BID × 7 days
   B. Azithromycin 1 g PO once + ciprofloxacin 500 mg BID × 5 days
   C. Ceftriaxone 250 mg IM once + azithromycin 1 g PO once
   D. Azithromycin 2 g PO once

5. Which of the following is the most appropriate second-line treatment option for this patient's diagnosis of chlamydia?
   A. Doxycycline 100 mg PO BID × 7 days
   B. Cephalexin 1000 mg PO BID × 7 days
   C. Levofloxacin 500 mg PO daily × 7 days
   D. Fluconazole 150 mg PO once

6. Which of the following is true regarding symptoms of chlamydia?
   A. Genital discharge is a cardinal symptom that is always present
   B. Many men and women are asymptomatic
   C. Men and women frequently complain of urinary retention
   D. Men and women complain of painful genital blisters

7. Regardless of recent sexual activity, how often should women under the age of 25 be screened for chlamydia?
   A. Every year
   B. Twice a year
   C. Every 3 years
   D. Only when symptomatic

8. Which of the following is true regarding gonorrhea and chlamydia infections?
   A. Partners of the co-infected individual only need to undergo treatment if intercourse occurred less than 60 days prior to the diagnosis of chlamydia and gonorrhea.
   B. Partners of the co-infected individual only need to undergo treatment if he/she is experiencing symptoms consistent with chlamydia or gonorrhea.
   C. Test-of-cure is not needed for persons with a diagnosis uncomplicated urogenital gonorrhea and chlamydia
   D. Test-of-cure is needed for all patients with co-infection of gonorrhea and chlamydia

9. Considering that this patient was initiated on azithromycin 1 g PO once, what would be the most important potential adverse reaction to include in your counseling session?
   A. Photosensitivity
   B. Edema
   C. Hyperglycemia
   D. Loose stools

ANSWERS

1. **Explanation:** The correct answer is A. Due to the TP's clinical findings of abnormal, odorless vaginal discharge, it is most likely that patient has gonorrhea (*N. gonorrhoeae*). Female patients infected with gonorrhea may complain of abnormal vaginal discharge or uterine bleeding as well as dysuria and urinary frequency.[1] Although the timing could be appropriate for syphilis/*T. pallidium* (10 to 90 days, mean 21 days), patients typically present with single, painless ulcer in the groin area.[1] Answers B and D are incorrect since a negative Whiff test and the absence of yeast reduce the likelihood of bacterial vaginosis (*G. vaginalis*) and vulvovaginal candidiasis (*C. albicans*), respectively. *G. vaginalis* is present in a diagnosis of bacterial vaginosis and patients typically have thin white or gray vaginal discharge in addition to pain, itching, burning, and a strong fish-like odor.[2]

2. **Explanation:** The correct answer is D. RPR card is used to screen for syphilis and serologic tests are used to detect blood antibodies against STIs such as syphilis, HIV, and hepatitis. Serology and RPR are not used for *N. gonorrhoeae* or *Chlamydia*. Wet mount/wet preparations of genital secretions are convenient and inexpensive and can provide clinicians with good insights regarding overall vaginal health; however, the sensitivity of vaginal specimen wet mount is low (51% to 65%). Nucleic acid amplification test (NAAT) such as polymerase chain reaction (PCR) can be performed on endocervical swab, vaginal swab, and

urine specimens and sensitivity is superior to cultures for diagnosing gonorrhea and/or chlamydia. NAATs offer a simplistic, efficient, and accurate testing option.[3]

3. **Explanation:** The correct answer is B. Due to the high frequency of *N. gonorrhoeae* and *Chlamydia trachomatis* (chlamydia) co-infection, treatment guidelines recommend that individuals treated for gonococcal infection also be treated with a medication regimen effective against uncomplicated *C. trachomatis* infection (this fact rules out answer choices A, C, and D).

4. **Explanation:** The correct answer is C. Answer A is incorrect since doxycycline alone does not provide good coverage for gonorrhea. Doxycycline may be used as a second-line agent to treat chlamydia. Fluoroquinolone-resistance against *N. gonorrhoeae* has been emerging in the United States over the past decade; therefore, the CDC no longer recommends using this class of antibiotics to treat gonorrhea (rules out answer B). Additionally, dual therapy has been recommended for the treatment of gonorrhea in order to improve treatment efficacy and slow any emergence of cephalosporin resistance. With this dual therapy recommendation, the CDC recommends using two antimicrobials with differing mechanisms of action with the primary agents being ceftriaxone and azithromycin. Oral cefixime and doxycycline may be alternatives to ceftriaxone and azithromycin, respectively. Answer choice D has had some clinical controversy recently since data has shown high effectiveness (approximately 99%) against uncomplicated urogenital gonorrhea; however, the treatment guidelines no longer support this regimen due to concerns regarding *N. gonorrhoeae* resistance against macrolides.[3]

5. **Explanation:** The correct answer is C. According to a meta-analysis consisting of 12 RCTs, azithromycin (recommend therapy) versus doxycycline for urogenital chlamydia treatment was shown to be equally efficacious; however, this patient has reported an allergy to doxycycline with lip and tongue swelling which makes it an inappropriate option (rules out answer A).[4] The extent of this allergy to doxycycline (swelling of lip and tongue) makes it an inappropriate option; therefore, it is important to collect accurate allergy history (timing and extent). Current guidelines endorse that levofloxacin (500 mg PO daily × 7 days) and ofloxacin (300 mg PO BID × 7 day) are effective treatments, although they may not be as cost-effective and offer no benefit regarding dosing regimen (Answer C). Additional alternative regimens include erythromycin 500 mg PO four times daily for 7 days or erythromycin ethylsuccinate 800 mg PO four times a day × 7 days.[3] Fluconazole is an antifungal and is effective against *Candida* infections (rules out answer D). Cephalexin is a first-generation cephalosporin and has poor coverage against intracellular bacteria such as chlamydia.[5]

6. **Explanation:** The correct answer is B. According to the current guidelines, asymptomatic infection is common among men and women, making screening an important aspect for diagnosis. Urethral and vaginal discharge may be present in persons with chlamydia but is more common with gonorrhea (rules out answer A).[3] Additionally, infected persons may complain of dysuria or urinary frequency rather than retention (rules out answer C). Painful genital blisters have not been associated with chlamydia and are more common in persons with genital herpes.[1]

7. **Explanation:** The correct answer is A. According the most recent guideline recommendations, annual screening is suggested for all women under the age of 25 years and for older women with increased risk (eg, more than one sex partners, sex partner with an STI, or those with a new sex partner) of infection (this recommendation rules out answer choices B, C, and D).[3]

8. **Explanation:** The correct answer is C. According to the most current guidelines, test-of-cure is not necessary for patients with uncomplicated diagnoses. Test-of-cure is recommended in certain situations such as pharyngeal gonorrhea, suspected treatment failure, special populations (pregnancy and neonatal), questionable adherence, and persistent symptoms among others (rules out answer D). Partners of infected persons should be referred for evaluation, testing, and treatment if sexual intercourse took place in the 60 days preceding the symptoms or diagnosis of chlamydia or gonorrhea, regardless of symptoms since many individuals are asymptomatic (rule out answer B). In the instance that the 60-day interval has passed, it is still recommended the most recent sex partner should still be evaluated and treated (rules out answer A). Although test-of-cure is not necessary, it is recommended that all men and women who have been treated for chlamydia or gonorrhea be retested roughly 3 months following treatment since reinfection may be present due to sexual partners neglecting to be treated or due to the individual engaging in sexual activity with a new infected partner. Regardless of if the person believes their sexual partner(s) were treated, retesting at 3 months is recommended.[3]

9. **Explanation:** The correct answer is D. According to drug information resources loose stools are a common and unfavorable occurrence with azithromycin use and the incidence may be higher with single-dose regimens. Photosensitivity is a potential adverse event with doxycycline, but the same risk is not present with azithromycin (rules out answer A). Answer choices B and C are potential counseling points, but these effects have less than 1% incidence and would not be the most important points to cover for single-dose regimens with azithromycin.[6]

REFERENCES

1. Knodel LC, Duhon B, Argamany J. Sexually transmitted diseases. In: Dipiro JT, Talbert RL, Yee GC, et al. *Pharmacotherapy: A Pathophysiologic Approach*. 10th ed. New York, NY: McGraw-Hill.

2. Hainer BL, Gibson MV. Vaginitis: Diagnosis and treatment. *Am Fam Phys.* 2011;83(7):807-815.

3. Workowski KA, Bolan GA. Sexually transmitted diseases treatment guidelines, 2015. *MMWR Recomm Rep.* 2015;64(No. 3):55-68.

4. Lau CY, Qureshi AK. Azithromycin versus doxycycline for genital chlamydial infections: a meta-analysis of randomized clinical trials. *Sex Transm Dis.* 2002;29(9):497-502.

5. Gallagher JC, MacDougall C. *Antibiotics Simplified*, 3rd ed. Sudbury, MA: Jones and Bartlett Learning.

6. Azithromycin. In: Wolters Kluwer Clinical Drug Information, Inc. (Lexi-Drugs); April 4, 2019.

28 Bacterial Vaginosis, Vulvovaginal Candidiasis, and Trichomoniasis

Elizabeth A. Cook   Jessica Wooster
Jonathan C. Cho

PATIENT PRESENTATION

Chief Complaint

"I'm having some issues with my private parts."

History of Present Illness

SP is 42-year-old Caucasian female presenting to her primary care provider for the above complaint. For the past seven days, she has experienced moderate vaginal discomfort, described as a burning/itching sensation around her vulvovaginal area, particularly when she urinates. She reports abnormal amounts of thin discharge from her vagina throughout the day. She is most perturbed by the odor and color of the discharge, which is dark yellow and foul smelling. She is recently divorced and is concerned that these symptoms will impact her social life, as she has began to experience pain during vaginal intercourse and is self-conscious of the odor of her discharge. Her last period was 2 weeks ago.

Past Medical History

T2DM, HTN, HLD

Surgical History

Adenoidectomy

Family History

Noncontributory

Social History

G3P2A1. Recently divorced after a 20-year marriage. Currently dating several men and has multiple male sexual partners. Does not use condoms during sexual intercourse. Denies tobacco use. Drinks 4 to 5 alcoholic mixed drinks on the weekends when out with friends.

Allergies

NKDA

Home Medications

Metformin 1000 mg PO BID W/F
Empagliflozin 25 mg PO daily
Lisinopril 20 mg PO daily
Atorvastatin 20 mg PO daily
Copper IUD inserted 2 months ago

Physical Examination

▶ **Vital Signs**

Temp 98.5°F, P 86 beats per minute, RR 16 breaths per minute, BP 124/72 mm Hg, pO_2 99%, Ht 5′8″, Wt 89.8 kg

▶ **General**

Slightly overweight, but well-groomed woman

▶ **Genital/Rectal**

Labia minora inflamed and red. No discharge issuing from urethra. Vagina exhibiting small amounts of frothy, thin yellow mucus, which emotes a putrid odor. Cervix completely visualized upon speculum insertion; appears pink with red "strawberry" lesions. Purulent discharge observed around endocervical canal.

Laboratory Findings

Na = 136 mEq/L	HbA1c = 6.8%
K = 4.1 mEq/L	TC = 126 mg/dL
Cl = 100 mEq/L	LDL = 68 mg/dL
CO_2 = 27 mEq/L	HDL = 54 mg/dL
BUN = 10 mg/dL	TG = 98 mg/dL
SCr = 0.6 mg/dL	
Glu = 106 mg/dL	
Ca = 9 mg/dL	

▶ *Urinalysis*

Color—light yellow, Clarity/turbidity—clear, pH—6, Specific gravity—1.005, Glucose—300 mg/dL, Blood—none, Ketones—none, Nitrites—negative, Leukocyte esterase—negative

▶ *Serum Pregnancy Test*

Negative

▶ *"Whiff" Test*

Negative

▶ *pH of Vaginal Secretions*

6

▶ *Vaginal Wet Mount*

Several motile pear-shaped, flagellating organisms, many leukocytes and minimal squamous epithelial cells are visualized in field. Clue cells and lactobacilli absent.

QUESTIONS

1. Based on the above signs, symptoms, and laboratory findings, which of the following conditions is/are most likely afflicting SP?
   A. Bacterial vaginosis
   B. Trichomonal vaginitis
   C. Vulvovaginal candidiasis
   D. Urinary tract infection

2. Which of the following pathogens is associated with causing the above diagnosis?
   A. *Gardnerella* sp.
   B. *Candida* sp.
   C. *Prevotella* sp.
   D. None of the above

3. Which of the following treatments would be most appropriate for treatment of SP's current condition?
   A. Clindamycin cream 2%, one full applicator PV QHS × 7 days
   B. Metronidazole gel 0.75%, one full applicator PV daily × 7 days
   C. Metronidazole 500 mg PO × 7 days
   D. Metronidazole 2000 mg PO × 1 day

4. Which of the following counseling points should be conveyed to individuals managed with the therapeutic agent selected above?
   A. Avoid drinking alcohol while actively taking this medication and for 24 hours following completion of therapy.
   B. Separate this therapy from foods, drinks, medications, and supplements containing polyvalent metallic ions.
   C. Sunscreen should be utilized while taking this treatment.
   D. Use of this medication may result in orange-red discoloration of feces, saliva, sweat, tears, and urine.

5. SP states that she has had sexual intercourse with several partners since symptom presentation 7 days ago. She is concerned that she may have transmitted her condition to these individuals. Which of the following statements/recommendations is true?
   A. Presumptive therapy should be initiated to all recent sexual contacts regardless of symptom presentation.
   B. Therapy should only be initiated if similar symptoms are present in the patient's sexual partners.
   C. This condition is not transmitted through sexual contact; thus, treatment is not required of sexual partners.
   D. This condition only manifests in female patients, thus only treatment of female sexual partners is required.

6. SP's primary care provider asks whether confirmatory testing for disease eradication will be necessary after completion of therapy. Which of the following monitoring plans is most appropriate?
   A. Confirmatory testing for disease eradication is recommended for both the patient and her sexual partners. Present to clinic within 3 months for follow-up.
   B. Confirmatory testing for disease eradication is only recommended for the patient. Present to clinic within 3 months for follow-up.
   C. Confirmatory testing for disease eradication is only recommended for patient's sexual partners. Present to clinic within 3 months for follow-up.
   D. Confirmatory testing for disease eradication is not warranted for the patient nor her partners.

7. SP calls your clinic 2 weeks later complaining of pruritus and erythema isolated to her vulvovaginal area. These symptoms are accompanied by scant vaginal discharge that is "thick and white like cottage cheese and doesn't smell bad like last time." She states that these symptoms are vastly different from those she experienced previously. She informs you that she has not had sexual intercourse since she saw you last month. Which of the following conditions is/are most likely afflicting the patient?
   A. Bacterial vaginosis
   B. Trichomonal vaginitis
   C. Vulvovaginal candidiasis
   D. Urinary tract infection

8. SP inquires whether there are any over-the-counter treatments that she can purchase at her local pharmacy to treat her new infection. Which of the following would be most appropriate over-the-counter treatment for SP's new condition?
   A. Clindamycin cream 2%, one full applicator PV QHS × 7 days
   B. Metronidazole gel 0.75%, one full applicator PV QHS × 5 days
   C. Miconazole 4% cream, once full applicator PV QHS × 3 days
   D. Terconazole 80 mg vaginal suppository PV QHS × 3 days

ANSWERS

1. **Explanation:** The correct answer is B. The patient's symptoms and laboratory findings do not align with vulvovaginal candidiasis, bacterial vaginosis, or a urinary tract infection (UTI), making trichomonal vaginitis the only correct answer. The odor and physical characteristics of her vaginal discharge, presence of cervical "strawberry spots" on her pelvic exam, vaginal pH, and flagellating protozoa visible in her vaginal wet mount are all supportive of a diagnosis of trichomonal vaginitis.[1] Uncomplicated UTI typically presents as lower urinary symptoms including dysuria, frequency, and urgency in otherwise healthy nonpregnant women.[2] Table 28.1 is provided below to compare and contrast characteristics of bacterial vaginosis, trichomonal vaginitis, and vulvovaginal candidiasis. The presence of the key characteristics listed in this table, are utilized by providers in the diagnosis and exclusion of common vaginal infections.[1]

2. **Explanation:** The correct answer is D. Trichomoniasis is associated with only one causative protozoan, *Trichomonas vaginalis*. *Gardnerella vaginalis* and other anaerobic bacteria (eg, *Bacteroides* sp., *Prevotella* sp., *Peptostreptococcus* sp.) are all common causative pathogens for bacterial vaginosis. *Candida* spp. are implicated in vulvovaginal candidiasis.[1]

3. **Explanation:** The correct answer is D. Only medications belonging to the nitroimidazole class (metronidazole and tinidazole) have activity against trichomonas. Therefore, clindamycin is not a viable option for the treatment of trichomoniasis, but is effective in the treatment of bacterial vaginosis. Nitroimidazoles have sufficient activity in eliminating anaerobic bacteria seen in bacterial vaginosis, which may demonstrate utility in the treatment of individuals presenting with both trichomoniasis and bacterial vaginosis. It is important to note that only oral nitroimidazole regimens are viable options for the treatment of trichomonas, as intravaginal metronidazole gel does not reach sufficient therapeutic levels in the urethra or perivaginal glands for full eradication. Additionally, oral metronidazole dispensed as a single-dose regimen should be the preferred treatment for trichomonal vaginitis, as several clinical trials have demonstrated its superiority in conveying parasitological cure compared to extended 7-day treatment regimens. Intravaginal metronidazole, which is effective in the treatment of bacterial vaginosis, is still considered a viable treatment option for that disease. Table 28.2 compares and contrasts the treatment of trichomoniasis and bacterial vaginosis to highlight potential errors that may occur in treating the two distinct conditions.[1]

4. **Explanation:** The correct answer is A. Alcohol consumption should be avoided during treatment with nitroimidazoles due to the potential for disulfiram-like reactions (eg, severe nausea and vomiting, flushing, tachycardia, hypotension). Due to the different half-lives of metronidazole and tinidazole, alcohol abstinence should be observed for 24 and 72 hours, respectively, after completion of therapy to ensure medication is eliminated from the body. Metronidazole does not chelate with polyvalent ions (eg, calcium, iron, magnesium), nor does it increase photosensitivity like tetracycline or quinolone antibiotics. Metronidazole use does not result in orange-red discoloration of body fluids,

TABLE 28.1. Characteristics of Vaginal Infections

Characteristic	Causative Pathogen		
	Bacterial	*Candida*	*Trichomonas*
Wet mount findings	Clue cells, minimal leukocytes	Mycelia fibers, minimal leukocytes	Pear-shaped, flagellating protozoa, increased leukocytes
pH	Elevated (>4.5)	Normal (3.5–5.0)	Elevated (>5.0)
Pelvic exam	Vulva and/or vagina may or may not be inflamed or erythematous. Abnormal volume of discharge is frequently present. Positive "whiff test".	Vulva and/or vagina is/are frequently inflamed or erythematous. Abnormal volume of discharge is frequently present.	Vulva and/or vagina may or may not be inflamed or erythematous. "Strawberry spots" visible on cervix. Abnormal volume of discharge may or may not be present.
Odor of discharge	Fishy	None	Malodorous
Color of discharge	Gray	White	White, yellow, or green-gray
Viscosity of discharge	Thin, homogenous	Thick, clumpy	Thick or thin, frothy

Source: Data from Workowski KA, Bolan GA; Centers for Disease Control and Prevention. Sexually transmitted diseases treatment guidelines, 2015. *MMWR Recomm Rep.* 2015 Jun 5;64(RR-03):1-137.

TABLE 28.2. Preferred and Alternative Regimens for the Treatment of Bacterial Vaginosis and Trichomoniasis

Treatment Regimens	Bacterial Vaginosis	Trichomoniasis
Preferred	Metronidazole 500 mg PO BID × 7 days OR Metronidazole gel 0.75%, one full applicator (5 g) PV once daily × 5 days OR Clindamycin cream 2%, one full applicator (5 g) PV QHS × 7 days	Metronidazole 2000 mg PO × 1 dose OR Tinidazole 2000 mg PO × 1 dose
Alternative	Tinidazole 2000 mg PO daily × 2 days OR Tinidazole 1000 mg PO daily × 5 days OR Clindamycin 300 mg PO BID × 7 days OR Clindamycin ovules 100 mg PV QHS × 3 days	Metronidazole 500 mg PO BID × 7 days

Source: Data from Workowski KA, Bolan GA; Centers for Disease Control and Prevention. Sexually transmitted diseases treatment guidelines, 2015. *MMWR Recomm Rep.* 2015 Jun 5;64(RR-03): 1-137.

TABLE 28.3. Over-the-Counter and Prescription Treatment Regimens for Vulvovaginal Candidiasis

Over-the-Counter	Prescription
Clotrimazole 1% cream, one full applicator (5 g) PV daily × 7–14 days OR Clotrimazole 2% cream, one full applicator (5 g) PV daily × 3 days OR Miconazole 2% cream, one full applicator (5 g) PV daily × 7 days OR Miconazole 4% cream, one full applicator (5 g) PV daily × 3 days OR Miconazole 100 mg one suppository PV daily × 7 days OR Miconazole 200 mg one suppository PV daily × 3 days OR Miconazole 1200 mg one suppository PV daily × 1 day OR Tioconazole 6.5% ointment, one full applicator (5 g) PV × 1 day	Butoconazole 2% cream (single dose bioadhesive product) 5 g PV × 1 day OR Terconazole 0.4% cream, one full applicator (5 g) PV daily × 7 days OR Terconazole 0.8% cream, one full applicator (5 g) PV daily × 3 days OR Terconazole 80 mg one suppository PV daily × 3 days OR Fluconazole 150 mg PO × 1

Source: Workowski KA, Bolan GA; Centers for Disease Control and Prevention. Sexually transmitted diseases treatment guidelines, 2015. *MMWR Recomm Rep.* 2015 Jun 5;64(RR-03):1-137.

as seen with agents such as rifampin, but does have the potential to cause brownish discoloration of the urine due to excretion of metabolites of the parent compound.[1]

5. **Explanation:** The correct answer is A. Presumptive treatment should be initiated in all sexual partners to prevent transmission or reinfection with *Trichomonas vaginalis* regardless of symptom presentation. Individuals should abstain from sexual intercourse until they and their partners have completed treatment and have achieved complete symptom resolution. Despite the name *Trichomonas vaginalis,* trichomoniasis can manifest in both females and males, so both sexes must be treated if they have engaged in intercourse with an infected individual. Males are frequently asymptomatic. If the patient had been infected with either bacterial vaginosis or vulvovaginal candidiasis, recommendations for the treatment of sexual partners differ. Evidence suggests that response to therapy and/or disease relapse remains unchanged when partners of women with bacterial vaginosis are provided with treatment. Therefore, presumptive treatment of bacterial vaginosis is not recommended. Additionally, uncomplicated vulvovaginal candidiasis is typically not transmitted through sexual intercourse and data do not support treatment of sexual partners.[1]

6. **Explanation:** The correct answer is B. Due to relatively high reinfection rates with *Trichomonas vaginalis,* up to

17% by some estimates, confirmatory testing for eradication is suggested for all females within 3 months following completion of initial treatment. Testing for disease eradication can be completed by wet mount, culture, enzyme immunoassay, nucleic acid probe test, or nucleic acid amplification. Data are currently insufficient to recommend retesting for males following completion of treatment for trichomoniasis. If not already performed at the initial visit, testing for other sexually transmitted diseases, including human immunodeficiency virus, should be completed by all parties. If the patient had been diagnosed with either bacterial vaginosis or vulvovaginal candidiasis, follow-up visits would not be considered necessary should her symptoms resolve following completion of medication therapy. Confirmatory eradication testing in females treated for either disease state has not shown evidence in reducing recurrence of uncomplicated infections or clinical outcomes. Additionally, follow-up testing would be considered unwarranted for partners considering sexual transmission is unlikely for both bacterial vaginosis and vulvovaginal candidiasis.[1]

7. **Explanation:** The correct answer is C. Based on the information provided by the patient, the most likely diagnosis is vulvovaginal candidiasis. The close proximity of her symptoms in relation to completing metronidazole therapy

may be indicative of an imbalance in normal vaginal flora, resulting in overgrowth of *Candida* sp. The signs/symptoms that the patient presents with do not correlate with her previous diagnosis of trichomonal vaginitis, making recurrent infection, or treatment failure, unlikely. The physical characteristics, absence of odor from the vaginal discharge, and lack of urinary symptoms also make it unlikely that the patient is presenting with bacterial vaginosis (Table 28.1). Uncomplicated UTI typically presents as lower urinary symptoms including dysuria, frequency, and urgency in otherwise healthy nonpregnant women, making this an unlikely diagnosis as well.[2]

8. **Explanation:** The correct answer is C. The preferred treatment of uncomplicated vulvovaginal candidiasis includes a short course of topical azole antifungal therapy, such as miconazole or terconazole. However, of those two agents, only the miconazole cream is available without a prescription. Table 28.3 highlights over-the-counter and prescription treatment modalities for vulvovaginal candidiasis. Of note, oral treatment with fluconazole is available, but requires a prescription. Both clindamycin cream and metronidazole gel would be effective in the treatment of bacterial vaginosis, but would not be effective in the treatment of vulvovaginal candidiasis. Furthermore, both the clindamycin cream and metronidazole gel would require a prescription to be dispensed to the patient for treatment.[1]

REFERENCES

1. Workowski KA, Bolan GA; Center for Disease Control and Prevention. Sexually transmitted diseases treatment guidelines, 2015. *MMWR Recomm Reports*. 2015 June 5;64(RR-03):1-137. Erratum in: MMWR Recomm Rep. 2015 Aug 28;64(33):924.
2. Gupta K, Hooton TM, Naber KG, et al. International clinical practice guidelines for the treatment of acute uncomplicated cystitis and pyelonephritis in women: a 2010 update by the Infectious Diseases Society of America and the European Society for Microbiology and Infectious Diseases. *Clin Infect Dis*. 2011;52(5):e103-e120.

29 Superficial Fungal Infections

Winter J. Smith   Jonathan C. Cho

PATIENT PRESENTATION

Chief Complaint

"I have an itchy rash on my stomach and feet that won't go away."

History of Present Illness

RP is a 16-year-old male who presents to his primary care provider's clinic at his mother's insistence because of a persistent pruritic rash on his trunk and feet. He is a high school sophomore and a member of the wrestling team. He reports having two areas on his trunk that are circular, red, and itchy. He says they have increased in size since he first noticed them about 3 weeks ago. He says his feet have always smelled bad, but he first started to notice redness and "extreme itching" between his toes on both feet about 2 weeks ago. He has used over-the-counter hydrocortisone cream on the rash on his trunk without improvement. He also started applying deodorizing spray to his feet a week ago without improvement.

Past Medical History

Seasonal allergies; asthma as a young child (asymptomatic for 10 years)

Surgical History

None

Family History

Father has diabetes, diagnosed at age 45; mother has HTN, diagnosed at age 38; both parents are living

Social History

Lives at home with parents and elder sister; denies tobacco, alcohol, and illegal drug use

Allergies

NKDA

Home Medications

Loratadine 10 mg PO daily
Occasional ibuprofen for muscle pain/sports injuries

Physical Examination

▶ **Vital Signs**

BP 118/78 mm Hg, P 60, RR 18 breaths per minute, Ht 5'11", Wt 82 kg

▶ **General**

Healthy-looking teenager, muscular build, well-developed, well-nourished, in NAD

▶ **HEENT**

Normocephalic, atraumatic, PERRLA, EOMI, moist mucous membranes

▶ **Pulmonary**

Normal breath sounds, no crackles or wheezes

▶ **Cardiovascular**

NSR, no m/r/g

▶ **Abdomen**

Soft, non-distended, non-tender, normal bowel sounds

▶ **Genitourinary**

Normal male genitalia without erythema or scaling

▶ **Neurology**

AAO × 4

▶ **Skin**

Two round, erythematous, and scaly areas visible on the trunk; each measures about 1 to 2 inches in diameter; each with a well demarcated, raised border and area of central clearing

▶ **Extremities**

Foul-smelling, dry, scaling feet with localized redness and white flaking between the toes. Toenails on both feet appear normal and without discoloration.

QUESTIONS

1. Which infections are consistent with RP's presentation? Select **ALL** that apply.
   A. Tinea capitis
   B. Tinea corporis
   C. Tinea cruris
   D. Tinea pedis
   E. Tinea unguium

2. What predisposing risk factor for infection does RP have?
   A. Age
   B. Male sex
   C. Contact sport
   D. Asthma history

3. Which empiric therapy is **most appropriate** for RP?
   A. Topical clotrimazole
   B. Oral terbinafine
   C. Topical nystatin
   D. Oral griseofulvin

4. Which is the most appropriate duration of empiric therapy for RP?
   A. 1 day
   B. 5 days
   C. 14 days
   D. 56 days

5. What is the goal of therapy for RP's infections?
   A. Negative fungal cultures
   B. Immune function restoration
   C. Resolution of systemic signs of infection
   D. Rash and symptom resolution

6. What nonpharmacologic measures can help prevent infection persistence/recurrence in RP? Select **ALL** that apply?
   A. Change socks every 3 days
   B. Wear the same shoes each day
   C. Keep affected body areas clean and dry
   D. Wear footwear in shared showers and locker rooms
   E. Share clothing and towels with teammates
   F. Wear absorbent socks

7. If RP completes his course of therapy but his infection persists without significant improvement, which is the **most appropriate** next step?
   A. Wait and watch, no antifungal therapy
   B. Topical antifungal therapy
   C. Oral antifungal therapy
   D. Intravenous antifungal therapy

8. Which infection would RP be at the highest risk for, in addition to his current infection, if he is not treated?
   A. Tinea capitis
   B. Tinea versicolor
   C. Tinea cruris
   D. Tinea unguium

ANSWERS

1. **Explanation:** The correct answers are B and D. Based on RP's complaints and the location of his symptoms, the most likely diagnoses are two different dermatophyte infections: tinea corporis (ringworm) and tinea pedis (athlete's foot).[1] In addition, the use of a topical steroid without symptom improvement suggests the presence of a superficial fungal infection. Tinea corporis generally appears as round, scaly lesions with a well-defined raised border and an area of central clearing. Use of topical steroids can alter the appearance of these lesions such that the central clearing and raised borders are not visible. This can make diagnosis difficult, and KOH microscopy may be needed for an accurate diagnosis. Tinea pedis often affects the skin between the toes, but can also impact other parts of the foot. Redness, flaking, and skin breakdown can also be observed. Despite the use of topical steroids, the characteristics of RP's trunk lesions and feet are classic presentations of tinea corporis and tinea pedis, respectively. Tinea capitis (answer A) is a dermatophyte infection of the scalp, tinea cruris (Answer C) affects the groin area (jock itch), and tinea unguium affects the toenails (onychomycosis). None of the other answer choices is consistent with RP's complaints or physical examination findings.

2. **Explanation:** The correct answer is C. Participation in contact sports is a well-known risk factor for dermatophyte infections due to close contact with other potentially infected athletes and the potential for transmission via surfaces and objects (eg, locker room floors, showers, towels, clothing, equipment).[1-4] Because of this, athletes should take precautionary measures to reduce the risk of infection and transmission.[2-4] Other risk factors for dermatophyte infections include excessive sweating (hyperhidrosis), living in close contact with others (eg, military housing), obesity, and diabetes.[5] Answers A and B are incorrect because tinea corporis and pedis can affect individuals of any age and sex.[1] (However, tinea capitis is most common in pediatric patients.[1]) RP's distant asthma history does not predispose him to dermatophyte infections (Answer D is incorrect).

3. **Explanation:** The correct answer is A. Topical antifungal agents are first-line for tinea corporis and tinea pedis cases that are not severe or extensive.[1] Topical options include azoles (eg, clotrimazole, miconazole, econazole), allylamines (naftifine, terbinafine), one benzylamine agent (butenafine), and one thiocarbamate agent (tolnaftate).[1,6] Most topical antifungal preparations are available without a prescription (over-the-counter [OTC]). Patients may select a specific formulation based on the site of infection, cost, and their preference.[7] Patients should be instructed to apply the selected product to the skin lesion(s) and one to two inches around the lesion(s).[7] Topical antifungal agents are well tolerated, only infrequently causing transient and mild skin irritation.[6] Although oral (systemic) terbinafine (Answer B) is effective against dermatophyte infections,

it is usually reserved for more severe/extensive infections or those that do not respond to topical therapy.[1,6] Another indication for systemic therapy, such as oral terbinafine and oral itraconazole, is fungal nail infections. Conventional topical antifungals do not penetrate the nail, and thus are not effective for treatment. Topical preparations designed specifically for fungal nail infections, such as ciclopirox, are also associated with low cure rates.[1] Answer C is incorrect because nystatin is ineffective against the organisms that cause dermatophyte infections. Nystatin is, however, an option for treating cutaneous *Candida* infections. Answer D, griseofulvin, is incorrect because topical therapy should be used first in this case. Also, oral griseofulvin requires longer treatment durations than many other oral antifungal agents used for dermatophyte infections. It is generally reserved for the treatment of tinea capitis.

4. **Explanation:** The correct answer is C. The frequency of topical antifungal application and duration of therapy vary based on the agent, but they are typically applied 2 to 3 times daily for 1 to 4 weeks.[1,6] While certain topical azole preparations may be effective after one day of treatment (Answer A) for vulvovaginal candidiasis, this is not the case for dermatophyte infections. Answer B is incorrect because the minimum duration of therapy is 7 days for topical terbinafine and 14 days for topical azoles.[1,6] It is important to note that the duration of therapy depends on the type of dermatophyte (tinea) infection as well as the severity and spread of the lesion(s). Answer D is incorrect for empiric therapy in cases that are not severe/extensive. However, longer durations of therapy may be necessary in cases that are severe/extensive, recurrent episodes, or do not respond to initial therapy.

5. **Explanation:** The correct answer is D. Tinea corporis and tinea pedis are most often diagnosed based on signs, symptoms, and physical examination.[1] Therefore, the goal/endpoint of therapy is clinical resolution (rash and symptoms). Answer A is incorrect, because cultures are not typically obtained for these infections. Answer B is incorrect because dermatophyte infections can occur in both immunocompetent and immunocompromised patients. The development of a dermatophyte infection does not provide information about a patient's immune function. Answer C is incorrect because RP has no systemic signs of infection, only local symptoms.

6. **Explanation:** The correct answers are C, D, and F. Cleaning the affected areas gently with soap and water as well as drying them thoroughly (Answer C) will help avoid the optimal environment for fungal growth (moist, warm).[2–4] Similarly, wearing absorbent socks (Answer F) can help keep the feet dry. Wearing footwear (eg, flip-flops) in shared showers and locker rooms (Answer D) can help prevent transmission via surfaces. Answer A is incorrect because socks should be changed at least daily. Answer B is incorrect, because shoes should be rotated daily to ensure that each pair dries completely before it is worn again.

Answer E is incorrect because sharing clothing and towels with teammates can promote the transmission of dermatophyte infections.

7. **Explanation:** The correct answer is C. Tinea corporis and tinea pedis infections that do not respond to initial topical therapy should be treated with oral (systemic) therapy.[1] Answer A is incorrect; oral (systemic) therapy is necessary if topical therapy fails. Answer B is incorrect because failure of topical therapy warrants the use of oral (systemic) therapy. Examples of oral therapy options for tinea corporis and tinea pedis include terbinafine 250 mg PO daily for 2 to 4 weeks, itraconazole 200 to 400 mg PO daily for 1 week (400 mg dose divided twice daily), and fluconazole 150 mg PO once weekly for 2 to 4 weeks.[6,8] Terbinafine is the most effective oral (systemic) therapy for onychomycosis treatment, with cure rates around 45%.[9] Common and significant side effects associated with terbinafine include headache, gastrointestinal (GI) disturbances, and hepatotoxicity.[6,8] Hepatic transaminase monitoring is recommended at baseline and periodically during therapy. Terbinafine use is not recommended in patients with liver disease or injury. Drug interactions are possible, as terbinafine is metabolized via CYP450 and is also a CYP2D6 inhibitor. Itraconazole (labeled indication) and fluconazole (off-label use) are less effective for the treatment of onychomycosis, with cure rates around 20%.[9] Itraconazole is available as an oral capsule (two formulations) and an oral solution.[6,8] The dosage form must be selected carefully due to differences in absorption. Itraconazole can cause GI disturbances, namely diarrhea and nausea, particularly in the oral solution form. Worsening of heart failure and new-onset heart failure have been reported with itraconazole use; it is contraindicated in patients with a history of heart failure. Itraconazole is both a substrate and an inhibitor of CYP3A4 and several drug interactions are possible. Like terbinafine, hepatic transaminase monitoring is recommended at baseline and periodically during therapy with itraconazole. Fluconazole is well tolerated with a low risk of liver toxicity.[6,8] With weekly dosing, fluconazole drug interactions are usually minimal.[6,8] Exceptions to this include narrow therapeutic index drugs like warfarin, phenytoin, and cyclosporine. Systemic azole antifungals (including itraconazole and fluconazole) are contraindicated in pregnancy, and treatment of onychomycosis in pregnancy is not recommended since therapy can be delayed until after delivery.[10] Breastfeeding should be avoided during terbinafine therapy. Answer D is incorrect; the next step after topical therapy failure is oral therapy, not intravenous therapy.

8. **Explanation:** The correct answer is D. Tinea unguium (onychomycosis) can develop as a result of untreated tinea pedis.[1] Onychomycosis often warrants oral (systemic) therapy and requires treatment for 3 to 6 months.[1,9] Alternatively, some milder cases of onychomycosis may be treated with topical antifungal preparations developed

specifically for nail infections (ie, not the same preparations used for cutaneous fungal infections). Answers A and C are incorrect. While different dermatophyte infections often coexist, as seen in this case, due to the proximity of the feet and toenails, RP is at highest risk of developing tinea unguium from untreated tinea pedis. Additionally, tinea capitis most often occurs in children. Answer B is incorrect because tinea versicolor (now named pityriasis versicolor) is a superficial fungal infection that is not considered a dermatophyte infection because it is not caused by a dermatophyte organism.[1] Dermatophytes are organisms in three genera, *Trichophyton*, *Microsporum*, and *Epidermophyton*. Pityriasis versicolor is caused by yeasts in the genus *Malassezia*.

REFERENCES

1. Ely JW, Rosenfeld S, Seabury Stone M. Diagnosis and management of tinea infections. *Am Fam Physician*. 2014;90:702-710.

2. Likness LP. Common dermatologic infections in athletes and return-to-play guidelines. *J Am Osteopath Assoc*. 2011;111:373-379

3. Centers for Disease Control and Prevention. Ringworm risk & prevention. Available at https://www.cdc.gov/fungal/diseases/ringworm/risk-prevention.html.

4. American Academy of Dermatology. Athlete's foot: How to prevent. Available at https://www.aad.org/public/diseases/contagious-skin-diseases/athlete-s-foot-how-to-prevent.

5. American Academy of Dermatology. Ringworm: Who gets and causes. Available at https://www.aad.org/public/diseases/contagious-skin-diseases/ringworm#causes.

6. Gupta AK, Cooper EA. Update in antifungal therapy of dermatophytosis. *Mycopathologica*. 2008;166:353-367.

7. PL Detail-Document. Topical antifungal agents for tinea infections. *Pharmacist's Letter/Prescriber's Letter*. May 2014.

8. PL Detail-Document. Comparison of therapies for onychomycosis. *Pharmacist's Letter/Prescriber's Letter*. May 2013.

9. Gupta AK, Versteeg SG, Shear NH. Onychomycosis in the 21st century: an update on diagnosis, epidemiology, and treatment. *J Cutan Med Surg*. 2017;21:525-539.

10. Pilmis B, Jullien V, Sobel J, Lecuit M, Lortholary O, Charlier C. Antifungal drugs during pregnancy: an updated review. *J Antimicrob Chemother*. 2015;70:14-22.

30 Cryptococcus

Paul O. Gubbins

PATIENT PRESENTATION

Chief Complaint

"My dad has been complaining of headaches and is now acting confused."

History of Present Illness

JK is a 68-year-old male, who was brought to the emergency department with a headache, nausea, and episodic vomiting that started about a week ago, and recent onset of dizziness, confusion, and irritability that was noticed today by his son while visiting with him for breakfast. He has a fever (101.3°F) of unknown duration. "A recent 4th generation HIV Ag-Ab test was negative." His son states that JK lives alone and started complaining of not feeling well about a week ago.

Past Medical History

Type 2 diabetes, controlled with medications

Surgical History

Appendectomy 20 years ago

Family History

Father had lung cancer and passed away 40 years ago; mother had HTN and passed away from stroke 15 years ago; no siblings

Social History

He is a retired salesperson, widowed (wife passed away from metastatic breast cancer 10 years ago), who lives alone. He has one son who visits him regularly. His hobby is golf and tending to a pet cockatoo; never smoked, but drinks alcohol occasionally

Allergies

NKDA

Home Medications

Metformin (Glucophage XR®) 2000 mg PO daily with evening meal
Multivitamin 1 tablet daily

Physical Examination

▶ **Vital Signs**

Temp 101.3°F, pulse 70, RR 20 breaths per minute, BP 130/92 mm Hg, pO$_2$ 92%, Ht 5′9″, 70 kg

▶ **General**

Lethargic, irritable gentleman with dizziness and confusion in moderate distress

▶ **HEENT**

Normocephalic, PERRLA, EOMI, (–) papilledema, photophobia, or blurred vision

▶ **Pulmonary**

Diminished breath sounds

▶ **Cardiovascular**

NSR, no m/r/g

▶ **Abdomen**

Soft, non-distended, non-tender, bowel sounds hyperactive

▶ **Genitourinary**

No complaints

▶ **Neurology**

Lethargic, oriented to place and person, (–) Brudzinski's sign, (–) Kernig's sign, (–) nuchal rigidity

▶ **Extremities**

Normal

▶ **Back**

Tenderness to palpation on lower lumbar region

Laboratory Findings

Na = 139 mmol/L	Hgb = 13.5 g/dL	Ca = 9.2 mg/dL	CK = 2.0 ng/mL
K = 4.2 mmol/L	Hct = 40%	Mg = 2.2 mg/dL	T Bili = 1.8 mg/dL
Cl = 100 mmol/L	Plt = 227	Phos = 4.4 mg/dL	Chol = 190 mg/dL

$CO_2 = 27$ mmol/L	WBC = 13.0×10^3	AST = 23 U/L	Trigly = 144 mg/dL
BUN = 40.0 mg/dL	Neut = 25%	ALT = 32 U/L	HDL = 54 mg/dL
SCr = 0.8 mg/dL	Lymphs = 70%	Alk Phos = 82 U/L	LDL = 90 mg/dL
Glu = 180 mg/dL	Monos = 5%	Tot Prot = 6.8 g/dL	BNP = 70 pg/mL

▶ Fourth-Generation Ag-Ab HIV

Negative

▶ CT Head

Unremarkable

▶ Blood Cultures

Pending

▶ Lumbar Puncture (LP)/CSF Analysis

CSF Glu = 35mg/dL	CSF Prot = 150mg/dL	CSF WBC = 13 (Neut = 20%; Lymphs 67%)

Crypto antigen—pending, opening pressure: 30 cmH_2O; Gram stain—no organisms observed; CSF cultures: pending.

QUESTIONS

1. What sign(s) or symptom(s) is/are characteristic of cryptococcal meningoencephalitis in JK?
   A. Nonspecific symptoms that developed over approximately a week
   B. The lack of an organism on CSF Gram stain
   C. The presence of CSF lymphocytic pleocytosis
   D. All of the above

2. What is the recommended initial antifungal induction therapy for JK?
   A. Amphotericin B deoxycholate 50 mg IV plus 5-FC 1,750 mg PO QID × 4 weeks
   B. Amphotericin B deoxycholate 50 mg IV plus fluconazole 800 mg PO daily × 2 weeks
   C. Amphotericin B deoxycholate 50 mg IV plus 5-FC 1,750 mg PO QID × 6 weeks
   D. Amphotericin B deoxycholate 50 mg IV plus fluconazole 400 mg PO daily × 2 weeks

3. How should increases in intracranial pressure be managed in JK during induction therapy?
   A. Administer mannitol 20 mg as an intravenous bolus dose
   B. Relieve by CSF drainage via lumbar puncture
   C. Administer acetazolamide 500 mg PO BID
   D. Administer prednisone 40 mg PO daily, and taper to response

4. How would recommended induction therapy differ from the case above if JK were a 35-year-old infected with HIV/AIDS diagnosed with cryptococcal meningoencephalitis?
   A. The duration of his induction therapy would be shorter.
   B. His induction combination therapy would include fluconazole instead of an amphotericin B formulation.
   C. His induction combination therapy would include an echinocandin instead of an amphotericin B formulation.
   D. He would receive fluconazole monotherapy as induction therapy instead of combination therapy.

5. Assume JK is a 35-year male with HIV/AIDS, diagnosed with cryptococcal meningoencephalitis and that he has successfully completed his induction and consolidation periods of treatment. What should be recommended for maintenance therapy?
   A. Fluconazole 200 mg PO daily indefinitely
   B. Itraconazole 400 mg PO daily indefinitely
   C. Fluconazole 200 mg PO daily for at least a year, then reassess based on HIV markers
   D. Itraconazole 400 mg PO daily for at least a year, then reassess based on HIV markers

6. How would recommended therapy differ from the case above if JK were a 40-year-old organ transplant recipient diagnosed with cryptococcal meningoencephalitis?
   A. He would receive an amphotericin B lipid formulation instead of the deoxycholate formulation.
   B. He would receive fluconazole as induction therapy instead of an amphotericin B lipid formulation.
   C. The duration of induction therapy would be prolonged.
   D. After completing consolidation therapy, JK would receive fluconazole 200 mg PO daily as primary prophylactic therapy indefinitely.

7. Which statement regarding the detection of relapsed infection is **TRUE**?
   A. Serial cryptococcal antigen testing should be performed to monitor therapeutic response and detect relapsed infection.
   B. Persistence of a positive CSF India ink stain is sufficient to detect relapsed infection.
   C. Detecting relapse only requires evidence of viable cryptococci from a previously checked sterile site.
   D. In detecting relapse, clinicians must assess the patient's adherence with consolidation or maintenance therapy.

ANSWERS

1. **Explanation:** The correct answer is D. Cryptococcal meningoencephalitis manifests as a subacute meningoencephalitis with nonspecific symptoms including fever, headache, lethargy, confusion, nausea, and vomiting that develop progressively over 1 to 4 weeks before a patient seeks medical attention. Although his presentation appears nonspecific, JK exhibits several findings including a CSF WBC <20/mm³, presenting with altered mental status, an opening pressure ≥25 cmH_2O, and hypoglycorrhachia

(a low CSF glucose level), that carry a poor prognosis. *Cryptococcus* possesses a capsule with immunosuppressive properties. It cannot be detected by Gram stain, but can be visualized with an India ink stain. The detection of *Cryptococcus* spp. by India ink stain is highly specific, but it is associated with a low sensitivity (≤50%). Therefore, serologic testing of blood and CSF should be done whenever cryptococcal CNS infection is suspected. Leukocyte count in the CSF is abnormally increased (lymphocytic pleocytosis), with a lymphocyte predominance.

2. **Explanation:** The correct answer is C. The correct dose for flucytosine (5-FC) is 100 mg/kg/d orally in four divided doses. Experts recommend at least 4 weeks for induction therapy for cases like JK.[1] However, the 4-week induction therapy (ie, initial therapy to reduce fungal burden) is reserved for cases with meningoencephalitis *without* neurological complications and cerebrospinal fluid (CSF) yeast culture results that are negative after 2 weeks of treatment.[1] JK has moderate evidence of neurological complications (eg, recent onset of dizziness, confusion, lethargy, and irritability) so the initial plan should be for 6 weeks of induction therapy. A reasonable approach in this case would be to reassess after 2 weeks of treatment by examining CSF yeast cultures and assessing clinical response (ie, improvement in symptoms, and laboratory findings, normalizing intracranial pressures). If cultures are negative and response excellent, clinicians in this case may opt to initiate consolidation therapy (ie, clearance of infected space) with fluconazole, while others may continue induction therapy for another 2weeks, shortening it from the initial plan of 6 weeks to a total of 4 weeks. Currently all induction regimens consist of 5-FC. If 5-FC cannot be administered (eg, significant myelosuppression, liver failure, renal failure, history of hypersensitivity), then induction therapy with amphotericin B monotherapy for a minimum of 6 weeks is warranted.[1] If JK had been AmBd intolerant in the past or had renal impairment, a lipid AmB formulation could have been used.

3. **Explanation:** The correct answer is B. Control of CSF pressure is a critical determinant of outcome for cryptococcal meningoencephalitis. Opening pressures in excess of 25 cmH$_2$O suggest a high fungal burden in the CSF and carry a poor prognosis. Thus, they must be addressed promptly. Mannitol has no proven benefit and should not be recommended.[1] Prednisone could be used to treat IRIS, which may occur in HIV-infected patients receiving highly active antiretroviral, but it has no role in treating increases in intracranial pressure in the absence of such symptoms. Similarly acetazolamide should be avoided as well.[1] Data in HIV-negative patients are sparse, but if the CSF pressure is ≥25 cmH$_2$O and the patient is symptomatic, CSF drainage via lumbar puncture should be performed to reduce the opening pressure by at least 50% if it is extremely high or to a normal pressure ≤20.[1] If elevations in intracranial pressure persist (ie, ≥25 cmH$_2$O), and the

patient is symptomatic, then daily lumbar puncture may be performed until the CSF pressure and symptoms have been stabilized for 12 days. In such cases, clinicians should consider temporary percutaneous lumbar drains or ventriculostomy (ie, a device that drains excess CSF from the head) for patient comfort. If these measures do not control increased intracranial pressure, then permanent ventriculoperitoneal (VP) shunts should be placed.[1]

4. **Explanation:** The correct answer is A. Given the lack of immune function and the likelihood of a large fungal burden in individuals with HIV infection, antifungal therapy should rapidly and consistently sterilize the CNS through rapid fungicidal activity. A sterile CSF culture 2 weeks after initiating therapy indicates a successful fungicidal induction regimen and is associated with favorable outcomes.[1] Several trials demonstrate the combination of amphotericin B formulations with 5-FC for 2 weeks of induction therapy produced the most rapid fungicidal effects and cleared the CSF significantly faster than other regimens, including amphotericin B deoxycholate monotherapy, or amphotericin B deoxycholate combined with fluconazole or therapy with all three agents together. Fluconazole is not an option for primary therapy due to a lack of fungicidal activity. Data demonstrate higher early mortality and reduced ability to clear the CSF rapidly with fluconazole alone. The echinocandins lack activity against *Cryptococcus neoformans*.

5. **Explanation:** Correct answer is C. Comparative trials clearly demonstrate that fluconazole is the most effective maintenance therapy.[1] In a clinical trial comparing fluconazole to itraconazole as maintenance therapy, fluconazole was proven superior. The trial was terminated prematurely after interim analysis revealed that significantly more itraconazole-treated patients had a relapse, compared to the fluconazole-treated patients.[1] Historically, life-long maintenance therapy to prevent disease relapse was recommended for all patients with AIDS after successful completion of primary induction therapy for cryptococcal meningoencephalitis. However, more contemporary data indicate the risk of relapse is low in patients meeting the following criteria: (a) They have successfully completed their primary therapy (including at least a year of maintenance therapy). (b) They remain asymptomatic and free of any signs of active cryptococcosis. (c) They are receiving highly active effective antiretroviral therapy, and their response to that has been stable [ie, a sustained CD4 cell count >100 cells/mL and an undetectable viral load (HIV RNA) for at least 3 months].

6. **Explanation:** The correct answer is A. In addition to CNS cryptococcosis, organ transplant recipients can develop pulmonary or disseminated infections. Regardless of the type of solid organ transplant, the immunosuppressive regimen following transplantation typically consists of a calcineurin inhibitor and approximately 25% of transplant

recipients have renal dysfunction when diagnosed. Thus, amphotericin B deoxycholate is not recommended as first-line therapy in this patient population. Fluconazole is not recommended for induction therapy. The lipid formulations are less potent on a weight basis, but are equally efficacious to the deoxycholate formulation when administered in recommended doses. Although most cases of cryptococcal disease in transplant recipients represent reactivation of an existing subclinical infection, such infections are difficult to detect and progress to disease in an unpredictable manner. Thus, routine prophylaxis for cryptococcosis in transplant recipients is not recommended.

7. **Explanation:** The correct answer is D. Serum and CSF cryptococcal antigen titers are important in establishing the presumptive diagnosis and assessing the prognosis of infection. The test measures cryptococcal polysaccharide capsule antigens, thus it does not differentiate viable from nonviable organism. CSF antigen titers are not precise indicators for early relapse or for making therapeutic decisions. Although serial antigen determinations are not useful, a single unchanged or rising CSF titer several months after initial diagnosis should raise clinical suspicion enough to warrant obtaining a culture. Similarly, India ink stain by itself is not sufficient for determining relapse, as the presence of lingering nonviable yeast in CSF is common. Positive India ink stains may be observed for up to a year following diagnosis despite treatment. Positive CSF culture for *C. neoformans* is diagnostic for microbiologic relapse or treatment failure. In order to detect relapse there must also be re-emergence of signs and symptoms at that infection site. In a relapsed infection, cultures and symptoms have normalized and then recurred. Most cases of relapse are due to inadequate primary therapy (dose and/or duration) or failure of compliance with consolidation or maintenance of fluconazole dose.

REFERENCE

1. Perfect JR, Dismukes WE, Dromer F, et al. Clinical practice guidelines for the management of cryptococcal disease: 2010 update by the Infectious Diseases Society of America. *Clin Infect Dis.* 2010;50:291-322.

31 Aspergillosis

Ashley H. Marx

PATIENT PRESENTATION

Chief Complaint

"I am coughing and very short of breath."

History of Present Illness

UL is a 47-year-old Caucasian male who presents to the emergency department via EMS with complaints of recent onset of fevers, shortness of breath, cough, and pleuritic chest pain. The patient reports that his symptoms began 3 days ago when he woke up in the middle of the night with shortness of breath and noticed sharp right-sided chest pain. The chest pain was provoked primarily by deep inspiration, and he was not able to go back to sleep. Last night, he began developing worsening chills, and also began to have wheezing and progressive shortness of breath. He also developed a productive cough, bringing up thick sputum eventually culminating in an episode of dry heaving and emesis. He states his emesis was originally dark blood, and toward the end of throwing up had some flecks of bright blood mixed in.

When EMS arrived at his home, UL was hypoxic (70% O_2 sat), tachypnic (RR 30), and tachycardic (HR 110s). He was administered nebulized albuterol and ipratropium and 1 L normal saline on the way to the hospital.

Past Medical History

Lupus erythematosus (inactive since 1992), coronary artery disease, deceased donor renal transplant 1994 secondary to lupus nephritis, CKD 4 (GFR 15-29); baseline SCR 2.5-3 mg/dL

Surgical History

Renal transplant 1994

Family History

Father has HTN and type 2 DM; mother alive and well

Social History

Married and lives with wife. No history of smoking or illicit drug use; drinks alcohol occasionally

Allergies

NKDA

Home Medications

Cyclosporine (Neoral®) 75 mg PO each morning, 50 mg PO each evening
Mycophenolate mofetil 500 mg PO twice daily
Prednisone 5 mg PO daily
Cholecalciferol (Vitamin D3) 1,000 units PO twice daily
Sodium bicarbonate 650 mg PO twice daily
Furosemide 20 mg daily as needed for swelling

Physical Examination

▶ Vital Signs

Temp 102.2°F, P 110, RR 24, BP 136/78 mm Hg, pO_2 95%, Ht 5'6", Wt 62.4 kg

▶ General

Middle-aged, thin gentleman in no acute distress

▶ HEENT

Anicteric sclera, pale conjunctiva, erythematous posterior oropharynx. Neck supple without lymphadenopathy

▶ Pulmonary

Inspiratory rales most prominent anterolaterally on both sides, few rales posteriorly

▶ Cardiovascular

NSR, no m/r/g

▶ Abdomen

Soft, non-distended, non-tender, bowel sounds present

▶ Back

No tenderness over renal allograft

▶ Genitourinary

Deferred

▶ Neurology

AO × 4

▶ Extremities

Normal, no lesions or edema

Laboratory Findings

Na = 136 mEq/L	Ca = 8.4 mg/dL	K = 4.1 mEq/L	Mg = 1.6 mg/dL
Cl = 107 mEq/L	Phos = 3.3 mg/dL	CO_2 = 21 mEq/L	AST = 23 IU/L
BUN = 45 mg/dL	ALT = 32 IU/L	SCr = 2.46 mg/dL	T Bili = 1.8 mg/dL
Glu = 88 mg/dL	Alk Phos = 130 IU/L	WBC = 8.2 × 10^3 mm^3	
		RBC = 2.19 × 10^3 mm^3	
Hgb = 6.7 g/dL	HCT = 20.0%	Plt = 33 × 10^3 mm^3	

▶ *Rapid Antigen Test*

Influenza negative; RSV negative

▶ *Legionella Urinary Antigen Test*

Negative

▶ *Chest X-ray*

Multifocal infiltrates, predominantly in the upper lobes. Bilateral pleural effusions

▶ *CT of the Chest*

Upper lobe predominant, groundglass and consolidative alveolar opacities bilaterally, left greater than right. Small bilateral pleural effusions

▶ *Initial Management*

UL is administered 1 unit PRBCs, lactated ringer's fluid 500 mL bolus × 1, then 100 mL/hr × 10 hours. Community-acquired pneumonia therapy was initiated with ceftriaxone 1 g IV plus azithromycin 500 mg IV daily. Based on UL's status as an immunocompromised host, a bronchoscopy was scheduled. Specimens from bronchoalveolar lavage (BAL) were sent for culture, galactomannan, *Mycoplasma pneumoniae* PCR, and direct fluorescent antibody (DFA) for *P. jirovecii*.

▶ *Bronchoscopy Results*

BAL gram stain: 1+ polymorphonuclear cells; no organisms
BAL culture: no growth
BAL galactomannan: 1.2 (normal <0.5)
DFA: negative for *P. jirovecii*
M. pneumoniae PCR: negative

Based on UL's compatible signs and symptoms, CT findings, and galactomannan result, he was diagnosed with probable invasive pulmonary aspergillosis. The decision was made to stop antibacterial therapy and initiate voriconazole 6 mg/kg IV q12h × 2 doses, followed by 4 mg/kg IV q12h. His mycophenolate will be stopped to lighten his immune suppression during this period of active infection. Assessment of clinical response and therapeutic drug monitoring will be guided by current national guidelines.[1]

QUESTIONS

1. Which risk factor for invasive pulmonary aspergillosis (IPA) is present in UL?
   A. High dose steroids for >1 month
   B. Solid organ transplantation
   C. Stem cell transplantation
   D. Environmental exposure from construction sites

2. Voriconazole was selected for therapy of invasive pulmonary aspergillosis. Voriconazole is likely to pose a significant drug interaction with which of his home medications?
   A. Cyclosporine
   B. Mycophenolate mofetil
   C. Furosemide
   D. Cholecalciferol

3. Assuming the patient clinically responds to therapy, what is the most appropriate minimum duration of therapy for treatment of IPA recommended in IDSA guidelines?
   A. 1 to 2 weeks
   B. 2 to 4 weeks
   C. 4 to 6 weeks
   D. 6 to 12 weeks

4. Which therapy is considered an alternative first-line therapy to voriconazole for the treatment of invasive aspergillosis?
   A. Caspofungin
   B. Itraconazole
   C. Isavuconazole
   D. Amphotericin B

5. For which antifungal(s) should therapeutic drug monitoring be recommended?
   A. Itraconazole
   B. Voriconazole
   C. Isavuconazole
   D. Both A and B

6. You are reviewing respiratory sputum culture results of a patient with cystic fibrosis who is currently experiencing an exacerbation. The most recent results are: 3+ methicillin-susceptible *S. aureus*, 3+ *Pseudomonas aruginosa*, and 1 colony of *Aspergillus fumigatus*. Which represents the best assessment and plan for this patient?
   A. Invasive pulmonary aspergillosis; initiate voriconazole
   B. Chronic necrotizing aspergillosis; initiate isavuconazole
   C. Allergic broncho-pulmonary aspergillosis; initiate itraconazole
   D. Possible *Aspergillus* colonization; do not initiate therapy

7. Which statement regarding antifungal susceptibility testing is true?
   A. Susceptibility testing is readily available and standardized in the same way as bacterial testing
   B. Susceptibility testing is available, but standardized interpretations are generally not

C. Susceptibility testing and interpretation is available only at reference labs

D. Susceptibility testing is not needed as resistance to antifungal drugs has not been described

8. Which are common adverse effects associated with voriconazole therapy?
   A. Visual disturbances and hepatotoxicity
   B. Neutropenia and nephrotoxicity
   C. Hypokalemia and hypomagnesemia
   D. Infusion-related reactions of fever and rigors

ANSWERS

1. **Explanation:** The correct answer is B, solid organ transplantation. Although UL has been on chronic steroids (which is an additional risk factor), his dose is not "high" or supra-physiologic at 5 mg daily. All listed choices are risk factors for the development of invasive pulmonary aspergillosis. Additional risk factors for IPA include chronic immune suppression (present in UL), hematologic malignancy, prolonged neutropenia, critical illness, hemodialysis, liver disease, COPD and other chronic lung diseases, and chronic granulomatous disease.

2. **Explanation:** The correct answer is A, cyclosporine. Voriconazole is metabolized by CYP4502C19, 2C9, and 3A4, and exhibits complex, dose-dependent drug interactions. Voriconazole is also a potent inhibitor of CYP450 3A4, which is involved in the metabolism of cyclosporine. Empirical reductions in cyclosporine doses of about 50% are recommended when voriconazole is initiated; this dose reduction should be recommended for UL. Significant drug interactions would not be predicted with furosemide, cholecalciferol, or mycophenolate, as none of these agents is metabolized by the CYP450 system.

3. **Explanation:** The correct answer is D. The minimum duration of therapy recommended for IPA is 6 to 12 weeks. In order to discontinue therapy, the patient should demonstrate good clinical response based on symptoms and radiographic improvement. Other durations listed are too short for invasive infection with *Aspergillus*. For UL, because he has an indication for on-going immune suppression, his course may be extended, or he may receive prophylaxis after active therapy. Another situation when prolonged therapy would be indicated would include dissemination to the central nervous system.

4. **Explanation:** The correct answer is C, isavuconazole. Isavuconazole was found to be non-inferior to voriconazole for the treatment of IPA. Amphotericin B is effective for the treatment of invasive aspergillosis, but is associated with significantly more adverse effects than azole therapy; further, amphotericin B formulations are associated with greater patient mortality due to IPA compared to voriconazole. As such, amphotericin B is considered a second-line therapy. Caspofungin, and other echinocandins, are used as salvage therapy (alone or in combination with other agents) for patients intolerant to or who have not responded to first-line

therapies. Itraconazole is effective for prophylaxis and treatment of less severe forms of aspergillosis such as brochopulmonary aspergillosis; however, it is not appropriate for invasive forms of aspergillosis.

5. **Explanation:** The correct answer is D. Both itraconazole and voriconazole exhibit significant intra-patient variability in serum concentrations, due to absorption (for itraconazole) and metabolism (for voriconazole). The recommended timing for concentration monitoring is within 60 minutes prior to the next dose (trough), usually after steady-state conditions have been reached. Therapeutic concentration ranges have been established for efficacy of itraconazole and voriconazole for the prevention and treatment of fungal infections; voriconazole toxicity is more often observed among patients with supratherapeutic concentrations. Relationships between isavuconazole concentrations and efficacy or toxicity have not been established, and therefore concentration monitoring is not recommended.

6. **Explanation:** The correct answer is D. Colonization of airways with environmental molds like *Aspergillus* is common, especially among patients with cystic fibrosis who cannot effectively clear respiratory secretions. The low quantity of mold in relation to high burdens of other common pathogens associated with cystic fibrosis exacerbations also support possible colonization. Choices A, B, and C represent diagnoses on the spectrum of diseases caused by *Aspergillus*, but signs and symptoms, and additional diagnostic tests would be required to establish one of these diseases.

7. **Explanation:** The correct answer is B. Antifungal susceptibility testing methods are described and must be validated according to the Clinical Laboratory Standards Institute in the United States; other regulatory bodies govern this process at international sites. The interpretation of susceptibility results is not as well-established as for bacterial pathogens, and breakpoints for susceptibility have been determined for relatively few pairs of fungal pathogens and drugs. Consultation with a microbiologist, infectious diseases specialist, and pharmacist is recommended when selecting therapy for clinical situations when breakpoints do not exist.

8. **Explanation:** The correct answer is A. Voriconazole causes visual disturbances, described as blurry vision or changes in color perception in up to 20% of patients. Up to 5% of patients experience hepatotoxicity. Choice B describes toxicities of flucytosine; choices C and D describe adverse effects of amphotericin B.

REFERENCE

1. Patterson TF, Thompson GRIII, Denning DW, et al. Practice guidelines for the diagnosis and management of aspergillosis: 2016 update by the Infectious Diseases Society of America. *Clin Inf Dis.* 2016;63(4):e1-60.

32 Protozoans

Lisa Avery

PATIENT PRESENTATION

Chief Complaint
Fever for almost a week

History of Present Illness
AB is a 58-year-old male with history of latent TB (s/p INH ×
9 months), recent month-long trip to Kenya, returned 1 week
ago and developed fevers, malaise, body aches, abdominal
pain, and headaches. He received multiple mosquito bites
while in Kenya, and did not take malarial prophylaxis. His
fevers occur every 24 to 48 hours.

Past Medical History
Hypertension, hyperlipidemia, diabetes, depression, latent
tuberculosis: s/p INH × 9 months

Surgical History
None

Family History
Father alive with type 2 diabetes, mother died at 72 of MI

Social History
Married with 2 adult children, nonsmoker, drinks occasionally

Allergies
NKDA

Home Medications
Citalopram 20 mg PO daily
Docusate 100 mg PO BID
Gabapentin 100 mg PO TID
Ibuprofen 400 mg PO q8h PRN fever
Lisinopril 20 mg PO daily
Acetaminophen 650 mg PO q6h

Physical Examination

▶ Vital Signs
Temp 103.3°F (oral), pulse 114 bpm, RR 18 breaths per min-
ute, BP 112/80 mm Hg (sitting position), SpO_2 97%, Ht 5'10",
Wt 87 kg

▶ General
Well-nourished, well-developed, patient appearing stated age
in no acute distress

▶ Eyes
Pupils equally round and reactive to light, no conjunctival
injection/scleral icterus, extraocular motions intact

▶ Ears/Nose/Throat/Mouth
Atraumatic external nose and ears. Moist mucous membranes; no pharyngeal erythema, no evidence of any
acute otitis media or external canal infection/mastoiditis
bilaterally. No nasal congestion noted. Neck: Supple and
non-tender. Trachea midline. No anterior cervical lymphadenopathy. No JVD

▶ Cardiovascular
Sinus tachycardia, no murmurs or gallops. Peripheral pulses
2+ and equal in all extremities

▶ Pulmonary
Unlabored respiratory effort. No wheezing, rhonchi, or rales
noted. No chest wall tenderness noted

▶ Abdomen
Abdomen is soft with nonspecific abdominal pain, is protuber-
ant and not distended. No masses or hernias appreciated. No
rebound, guarding, or peritoneal signs noted. Splenomegaly
present.

▶ Musculoskeletal
Extremities without deformity, edema or tenderness to
palpation

▶ Skin
Warm, dry; no rashes or lesions

▶ Neurological
Normal gait and balance; sensation grossly intact

▶ Psychiatric
Awake, alert, and oriented to date and time and person; appropriate mood and affect

Laboratory Findings

Na = 134 mEq/L	Hgb = 12.6 g/dL	Ca = 8.4 mg/dL
K = 3.9 mEq/L	Hct = 46%	Mg = 2.2 mg/dL
Cl = 98 mEq/L	Plt = 25×10^3 /mm³	Phos = 4.6 mg/dL
CO_2 = 24 mEq/L	WBC = 2.5×10^3 mm³	AST = 51 IU/L
BUN = 16 mg/dL	MCV = 81.6 L/cell	ALT = 109 IU/L
SCr = 0.86 mg/dL	MCH = 27 g/cell	T Bili = 2.6 mg/dL
Glu = 364 mg/dL	MCHC = 33 g/L	Alk Phos = 223 IU/L
A1C = 14.3%	PT = 10.3	Albumin = 2.5 g/dL
Lactate = 2.13	aPTT = 28.5	
Lipase = 226	D-dimer = negative	

▶ Chest X-ray

No acute disease

▶ Microscopic Examination of Blood

Peripheral smear under microscopy shows ring forms

▶ Blood Parasite

Plasmodium falciparum parasitemia 2.5%

▶ HIV Test

Nonreactive

▶ EKG

QTc = 492 ms

QUESTIONS

1. Which clinical symptoms are consistent with the diagnosis of malaria?
   A. Fever
   B. Muscle aches
   C. Abdominal pain
   D. All of the above

2. Which of the following laboratory tests are consistent with the diagnosis of malaria?
   A. Leukopenia, hyperglycemia, and hypokalemia
   B. Elevated hepatic enzymes, thrombocytopenia, and anemia
   C. Macrocytic anemia
   D. Elevated bicarbonate and elevated lactate

3. Which of the following statements are true regarding this patient's disease severity?
   A. This patient is asymptomatic and does not require any treatment
   B. This patient has uncomplicated disease and should be treated with oral therapy
   C. This patient has severe disease and should be treated with intravenous therapy
   D. The treatment is the same and does not depend on the severity of illness.

4. Which of the following statement is TRUE regarding *Plasmodium falciparum*?
   A. It causes a rapidly progressive disease
   B. The dormant form remains in the liver and causes relapsing disease
   C. There is little reported resistance to commonly prescribed medications
   D. It is not detected with rapid malaria diagnostic tests

5. AB recently traveled to Kenya where there is chloroquine resistance. Based on his disease severity, species, and potential resistance what would be the most appropriate therapy?
   A. Atovaquone-proguanil (250 mg/100 mg) 4 tablets PO daily × 3 days + primaquine phosphate 30 mg base PO daily × 14 days
   B. Hydroxychloroquine 620 mg base PO × 1, then 310 mg base PO at 6, 24, and 48 hours. Total dose = 1550 mg base
   C. Artemether-lumefantrine (20 mg/120 mg) 4 tablets, repeat 8 hours later, then twice daily × 2 days
   D. Atovaquone-proguanil 250 mg/100 mg 4 tablets PO daily x 3 days

6. AB's 22-week pregnant daughter is planning a trip to Kenya in 2 weeks. What would be the most appropriate malaria chemoprophylaxis regimen?
   A. Atovaquone-proguanil 1 tablet daily, start 1 to 2 days before traveling
   B. Doxycycline 100 mg PO daily, start 1 to 2 days before traveling
   C. Mefloquine 228 mg base weekly, start 1 to 2 weeks before traveling
   D. Tafenoquine 200 mg PO weekly, start 3 days before traveling

7. In addition to chemoprophylaxis, what nonpharmacologic measures can be employed to decrease AB's daughter's risk of malaria transmission?
   A. Pure oil of lemon eucalyptus on skin not covered by clothing
   B. DEET on skin not covered by clothing
   C. Permethrin directly on skin
   D. Since she is pregnant she should NOT use any insect repellants

ANSWERS

1. **Explanation:** The correct answer is D. Adult patients who present with malaria may present with nonspecific symptoms, which include fever, muscle aches, and

abdominal pain (nausea, vomiting, and diarrhea). These symptoms are characteristic of uncomplicated diseases.[1] Severe malaria or complicated disease occurs when the diseases progress to involve organ dysfunction including neurologic symptoms (dizziness, confusion, disorientation, seizures, and coma), acute respiratory distress syndrome, and renal dysfunction, which can be permanent. The typical incubation period for *P. falciparum* is 10 to 14 days, which coincides with this patient's return from Kenya 1 week ago. The fever associated with malaria typically includes high fever, shaking chills, and sweats (paroxysm) and can every 24 to 72 hours be dependent on the parasite species. These fever spikes correspond to the burst of red blood cells and the release of parasites into the bloodstream.

2. **Explanation:** The correct answer is B. In most cases hepatic enzymes will be elevated with thrombocytopenia common in uncomplicated malaria. Patients with a normal platelet count should be evaluated for an alternative diagnosis. Patients may also experience a normochromic, normocytic anemia as seen in this patient. This is secondary to red blood cell hemolysis in addition to decreased production of erythropoietin. Patients with severe disease may experience acidosis with a compensatory decrease in bicarbonate. Hypoglycemia may occur, although this is more common in children.

3. **Explanation:** The correct answer is B. It is important to classify the severity of illness to help determine whether intravenous or oral therapy is necessary. If a patient has one or more of the following criteria, he/she would have severe disease and would require hospitalization and intravenous therapy. Severe malaria is a medical emergency and requires prompt and aggressive treatment.[2]

- Impaired consciousness or coma
- Severe normocytic anemia (hemoglobin <7 g/dL)
- Renal failure
- Acute respiratory distress syndrome (ARDS)
- Hypotension
- Disseminated intravascular coagulation (DIC)
- Spontaneous bleeding
- Acidosis
- Hemoglobinuria
- Jaundice
- Repeated convulsions
- Parasitemia ≥5%

This patient does not meet any of the above criteria for severe disease and is diagnosed with uncomplicated disease. He should receive oral therapy. The clinical symptoms associated with uncomplicated disease are generally nonspecific and may be confused with the common cold. That is why an accurate travel history is important in nonendemic regions.

4. **Explanation:** The correct answer is A. Both *P. falciparum* and *P. knowles* are associated with rapidly progressive, severe disease if not treated promptly. *P vivax* and *P. ovale* have intrahepatic forms that may remain dormant as hypnozoites anywhere from 2 weeks to greater than 1 year and may cause relapses. It is important to check the resistance patterns for *P. falciparum* and *P. vivax* since there are different patterns of resistance depending on the geographically region where the patient was infected. Current rapid diagnostic testing (Binax Now) does detect *P. falciparum* since it detects histidine-rich protein-2 antigen that is specific to *P. falciparum* in addition to a common malaria antigen.

5. **Explanation:** The correct answer is D. This patient has uncomplicated malaria with *P. falciparum* in an area with chloroquine resistance. The CDC malaria guidelines recommend atovaquone-proguanil, arthemether-lumefantrine oral, quinine sulfate in combination with doxycycline, tetracycline, or clindamycin, or mefloquine monotherapy as treatment options for this patient.[2] Artemether-lumefantrine is considered first-line therapy per the 2015 WHO guidelines, but would not be an appropriate choice in this patient since it is associated with QTc prolongation and the patient has an elevated QTc, electrolyte abnormalities, and is on concomitant citalopram.[3] Quinine is also associated with QTc prolongation. Mefloquine would also not be an optimal choice, since this patient has active depression. Mefloquine can cause severe anxiety, paranoia, hallucinations, depression, restlessness, and unusual behavior. Atovaquone-proguanil would be the correct answer and needs to be taken with food or whole milk to increase absorption and decrease adverse reactions. The most common adverse reactions are stomach pain, nausea, vomiting, and headache. If the patient vomits within 30 minutes of the dose, repeat dose. The addition of primaquine phosphate is not necessary for this patient; since it treats the dormant hypnozoites in the liver that occurs with *P vivax* or *P. ovale* infections. Hydroxychloroquine is used only in the treatment of chloroquine-sensitive isolates.

6. **Explanation:** The correct answer is C. Mefloquine can be used during pregnancy and should be started 1 to 2 weeks before departure and continued for 4 weeks after leaving Kenya. None of the other choices can be used during pregnancy. AB should contact her physician if she experiences signs of severe anxiety, feelings of mistrust toward others, seeing or hearing things that are not present, depression, restlessness, or confusion. The most common side effects include nausea, vomiting, diarrhea, abdominal pain, dizziness, headache, and sleeping problems.

7. **Explanation:** The correct answer is B. Pregnant women can use insect repellants approved by the Environmental Protection Agency (EPA). DEET has been approved. The CDC recommends DEET concentrations greater than or equal to 20%.[4] If the concentration is less than 10%, there is only 1 to 2 hours of protection. Concentrations greater

than 50% provide no further benefit. Pure oil of lemon eucalyptus has not been tested by the EPA and should not be used. Permethrin should not be used directly on the skin, it should be sprayed on clothing as another line of defense against mosquitoes.[3] Counseling points for DEET application include the following: apply repellent only to exposed skin or clothing, do not apply under-clothing, do not use on open skin, do not apply directly on face, wash hands after application, heavy application of repellent does not improve efficacy, and after returning indoors wash skin thoroughly with soap and water.

REFERENCES

1. Centers for Disease Control and Prevention. Malaria. Available at https://www.cdc.gov/parasites/malaria/index.html. Accessed September 26.

2. Centers for Disease Control and Prevention. Guidelines for treatment of malaria in the United States. Available at https://www.cdc.gov/malaria/resources/pdf/Treatment-Table_2018.pdf. Accessed September 26.

3. World Health Organization. *Guidelines for the Treatment of Malaria*. 3rd ed. Available at https://www.who.int/malaria/publications/atoz/9789241549127/en/. April 2015. Accessed September 26.

4. Centers for Disease Control and Prevention. Insect repellents help prevent malaria and other diseases spread by mosquitoes. Available at https://www.cdc.gov/malaria/resources/pdf/fsp/repellents_2015.pdf. Accessed September 26.

33 Nematodes

Jessica Robinson

PATIENT PRESENTATION

Chief Complaint
Restlessness at night

History of Present Illness
LT is a 5-year-old male who presents to your clinic today for a wellness check. His mother states that over the last week he has been restless while sleeping. Otherwise, LT is healthy. While giving him a bath, she has noted mild perianal irritation but no change in bowel frequency or diarrhea. LT has complained of being "itchy" at night on several occasions, but has no other complaint. He has no recent history of travel or walking barefoot, and the family currently does not own pets. There has been no change in laundry detergent or introduction of new fabrics or soaps. LT's mother is not overly concerned but does want to ensure nothing is wrong.

Past Medical History
Seasonal allergic rhinitis

Surgical History
Tympanostomy tube placement

Family History
Mother has depression; father has type 1 DM; sister (age 3) is healthy

Social History
Mother reports he eats a balanced diet and is active throughout the day.

Allergies
NKDA

Home Medications
Loratadine 5 mg PO daily

Physical Examination

▸ **Vital Signs**

Temp 98.1°F, P 95 bpm, RR 22 breaths per minute, BP 100/60 mm Hg, Ht 3'2", Wt 19 kg

▸ **General**

Energetic, talkative 5-year old in no obvious distress

▸ **HEENT**

Normocephalic, atraumatic, PEERLA, good dentition

▸ **Pulmonary**

Lungs clear, no abnormal breath sounds

▸ **Cardiovascular**

NSR, no m/r/g

▸ **Abdomen**

Soft, non-distended, non-tender, bowel sounds normal

▸ **Genitourinary**

Normal male genitalia, scratch marks present near rectum

▸ **Neurology**

Oriented to person, place, time

▸ **Extremities**

Range of motion intact, no evidence of skin rashes

Laboratory Findings

Na: 138 mEq/L	Hgb: 14.5 g/dL
K: 4.1 mEq/L	Hct: 37%
Cl: 105 mEq/L	Plt: $200 \times 10^3/mm^3$
CO_2: 25 mEq/L	WBC: $7.2 \times 10^3/mm^3$
Glucose: 68 mg/dL	
SCr: 0.6 mg/dL	
BUN: 10 mg/dL	

QUESTIONS

1. What is the likely cause of LT's infection?
   A. Ascariasis
   B. Strongyloidiasis
   C. Hookworm disease
   D. Enterobiasis

2. What diagnostic testing and/or imaging will be the most helpful in confirming this diagnosis?
   A. Microscopic examination of stool
   B. Cellulose acetate tape test
   C. Abdominal X-ray
   D. Abdominal CT

3. What is the most appropriate initial drug therapy for LT?
   A. Albendazole
   B. Itraconazole
   C. Praziquantel
   D. Metronidazole

4. What special instructions should be given when prescribing albendazole for pinworm infection?
   A. Take it with an acidic beverage to facilitate absorption.
   B. Recommend a dose now, and a second dose 2 weeks later.
   C. This mediation cannot be crushed.
   D. Counsel on the severe gastrointestinal side effects often seen with this medication.

5. LT and his sister co-sleep several nights a week. She is currently not exhibiting any signs or symptoms of illness, but her mother is concerned she could also be infected. What is the most appropriate recommendation?
   A. Do not treat her at this time, pinworm infection is generally not contagious.
   B. Do not treat her at this time, you only treat patients if they are symptomatic.
   C. Treat her today with albendazole, pinworm infections are highly contagious and it is generally advisable to treat all members of the household.
   D. Treat her today with albendazole, pinworm infections may be contagious, but because she co-sleeps with LT she is likely infected.

6. LT's mother is currently pregnant with her third child (2nd trimester). She also reports no current symptoms of infection. Would you recommend treatment for her?
   A. Yes, recommend treatment with albendazole.
   B. Yes, recommend treatment with mebendazole.
   C. Yes, recommend treatment with pyrantel pamoate.
   D. No, do not recommend treatment at this time.

7. Which of the following environmental precautions should not be recommended?
   A. Shower every night to help prevent the spread of pinworm and to prevent reinfection.
   B. Follow good hand hygiene practices, especially after using the bathroom.
   C. Avoid biting fingernails and be sure to cut fingernails regularly.
   D. Wash all clothes and bedding each morning in hot water.

ANSWERS

1. **Explanation:** The correct answer is D. The most common manifestation of enterobiasis, or pinworm, infection is perianal irritation.[1,2] This is often the only symptom. Ascariasis, strongyloidiasis, and hookworm disease are often asymptomatic. Ascariasis does have the potential to cause gastrointestinal or pulmonary symptoms. Strongyloidiasis may cause abdominal pain similar to that of a peptic ulcer, but can disseminate to other organ systems. Hookworm may also cause gastrointestinal symptoms, and chronic infection may cause iron deficiency anemia.[2]

2. **Explanation:** The correct answer is B. While microscopic examination of stool is the preferred diagnostic method for other infections caused by nematodes, pinworms are not released in the feces. Therefore, cellulose acetate tape must be applied to the rectum and examined microscopically to detect the presence of eggs. Abdominal images have no role in diagnosis.[2]

3. **Explanation:** The correct answer is A. Three treatment options currently exist for enterobiasis: albendazole, mebendazole, and pyrantel pamoate.[1,2] All are given initially as one-time doses. Albendazole (dosed as 200 mg PO × 1 in children <2 years, 400 mg PO × 1 in children >2 years) and mebendazole (100 mg PO × 1) are available only via prescription (mebendazole is only available from compounding pharmacies in the United States), while pyrantel pamoate (11 mg/kg PO × 1) is available over the counter.[3] Itraconazole, praziquantel, and metronidazole have no role in therapy for pinworm infection.

4. **Explanation:** The correct answer is B. Albendazole should be given as a one-time dose now, and then again 2 weeks later due to concern for reinfection, as albendazole does not reliably kill pinworm eggs and a second dose can kill any adult worms that have hatched after the initial treatment. Albendazole can be crushed if the child is unable to swallow pills.[3] It is generally very well tolerated.

5. **Explanation:** The correct answer is C. It is generally recommended to treat all household members if one has been diagnosed with a pinworm infection. While you may withhold treatment in certain situations, most health care professionals will treat the entire household at one time to prevent reinfection.[1] Medications for the treatment of pinworm are generally safe and well-tolerated.

6. **Explanation:** The correct answer is D. All three agents are pregnancy category C. As per CDC recommendations, a woman may be treated in the third trimester if the infection is complicating the pregnancy. Otherwise, these medications should be avoided due to lack of safety data in pregnant patients.[1]

7. **Explanation:** The correct answer is A. Once ingested, pinworms migrate to the colon and lay eggs around the anus at night. Therefore, it is best to take a shower each morning to wash away any eggs that may be present. All clothing and bedding should also be washed in the morning. Because perianal irritation is common, eggs may be present under the fingernails due to scratching. Therefore, it is important to not bite fingernails to prevent any possible reinfection. Appropriate hand hygiene is always recommended.[1]

REFERENCES

1. Centers for Disease Control and Prevention. Enterobiasis. Available at https://www.cdc.gov/parasites/pinworm/. Accessed September 27, 2019.

2. Weller PF, Nutman TB. Intestinal nematode infections. In: Jameson J, Fauci AS, Kasper DL, Hauser SL, Longo DL, Loscalzo J, eds. *Harrisons Principles of Internal Medicine*, 20 ed. New York, NY: McGraw-Hill. Available at http://accessmedicine.mhmedical.com/content.aspx?bookid=2129&sectionid=192027581. Accessed September 27, 2019.

3. Lexicomp Online. *Pediatric Drug Information*. Hudson, OH: Wolters Kluwer Clinical Drug Information; 2019.

34 Tuberculosis

David Cluck

PATIENT PRESENTATION

Chief Complaint

"I have a cough that won't go away."

History of Present Illness

A 63-year-old male presents to the emergency department with complaints of cough/shortness of breath which he attributes to a "nagging cold." He states he fears this may be something worse after experiencing hemoptysis for the past 3 days. He also admits to waking up in the middle of the night "drenched in sweat" for the past few weeks. When asked, the patient denies ever having a positive PPD and was last screened "several years ago." His chart indicates he was in the emergency department last week with similar symptoms and was diagnosed with community-acquired pneumonia and discharged with azithromycin.

Past Medical History

Hypertension, dyslipidemia, COPD, atrial fibrillation, generalized anxiety disorder

Surgical History

Appendectomy at age 18

Family History

Father passed away from a myocardial infarction 4 years ago; mother had type 2 DM and passed away from a ruptured abdominal aortic aneurysm

Social History

Retired geologist recently moved from India to live with his son who is currently in medical school in upstate New York. Smoked ½ ppd × 40 years and drinks 6 to 8 beers per day, recently admits to drinking ½ pint of vodka "every few days" since the passing of his wife 6 months ago.

Allergies

Sulfa (hives); penicillin (nausea/vomiting); shellfish (itching)

Home Medications

Albuterol metered-dose-inhaler 2 puffs q4h PRN shortness of breath

Aspirin 81 mg PO daily
Atorvastatin 40 mg PO daily
Budesonide/formoterol 160 mcg/4.5 mcg 2 inhalations BID
Clonazepam 0.5 mg PO three times daily PRN anxiety
Lisinopril 20 mg PO daily
Metoprolol succinate 100 mg PO daily
Tiotropium 2 inhalations once daily
Venlafaxine 150 mg PO daily
Warfarin 7.5 mg PO daily

Physical Examination

▶ **Vital Signs**

Temp 100.8°F, P 96, RR 24 breaths per minute, BP 150/84 mm Hg, pO_2 92%, Ht 5'10", Wt 56.4 kg

▶ **General**

Slightly disheveled male in mild-to-moderate distress

▶ **HEENT**

Normocephalic, atraumatic, PERRLA, EOMI, pale/dry mucous membranes and conjunctiva, poor dentition

▶ **Pulmonary**

Bronchial breath sounds in RUL

▶ **Cardiovascular**

NSR, no m/r/g

▶ **Abdomen**

Soft, non-distended, non-tender, (+) bowel sounds

▶ **Genitourinary**

No complaint of dysuria or hematuria

▶ **Neurology**

Oriented to person, place, and time

▶ **Extremities**

No lesions or edema present

Laboratory Findings

Na = 140 mEq/L   Hgb = 14.5 g/dL   Ca = 8.8 mg/dL

K = 4.5 mEq/L   Hct = 38%   Mg = 2.2 mg/dL

Cl = 98 mEq/L   Plt = 332 × 10³/mm³ Phos = 4.6 mg/dL

CO_2 = 26 mEq/L   WBC = 12 × 10³ mm³   AST = 24 IU/L

BUN = 26 mg/dL   Trop <0.01 ng/mL   ALT = 22 IU/L

SCr = 1.48 mg/dL   CK = 3 ng/mL   T Bili = 1.8 mg/dL

Glu = 188 mg/dL   BNP = 64 pg/mL   Alk Phos = 76 IU/L

INR = 2.4

► Chest X-ray

Hilar lymphadenopathy visualized with RUL apical and posterior segment infiltrate

► Blood Culture

Negative

► Sputum Culture

Normal flora

► Sputum AFB Culture

Pending

► Influenza Screen

Negative

QUESTIONS

1. Which risk factor places this patient at highest risk of developing tuberculosis disease?
   A. Being foreign born
   B. Failure of CAP treatment
   C. Hemoptysis
   D. History of COPD

2. Which diagnostic criteria would suggest highest likelihood of tuberculosis disease?
   A. Positive AFB sputum smears plus negative NAA
   B. Positive IGRA only
   C. Positive IGRA plus chest radiography
   D. Positive AFB sputum smear plus positive NAA

3. Which empiric regimen is most appropriate for active tuberculosis disease?
   A. Ethambutol plus clarithromycin
   B. Rifapentine plus isoniazid
   C. Rifabutin plus ethambutol
   D. Rifampin plus ethambutol plus pyrazinamide plus isoniazid

4. In a fully active tuberculosis regimen, which agent may be discontinued if the organism is susceptible to all first-line agents?
   A. Ethambutol
   B. Isoniazid

C. Pyrazinamide
D. Rifampin

5. The patient is started on a regimen of rifampin/ethambutol/pyrazinamide/isoniazid (RIPE). Shortly after starting his therapy the patient presents to an urgent care with concern his "blood is too thin" due to overt red-tinged urine; however, a urinalysis is negative for blood. The provider recognizes the drug–drug interaction with warfarin and rifampin and asks for a recommendation to manage this drug–drug interaction. Which recommendation is most appropriate?
   A. Switch warfarin to rivaroxaban
   B. Continue warfarin with close monitoring
   C. Switch rifampin to rifapentine
   D. Add enoxaparin while taking rifampin

6. Three weeks into therapy his liver enzymes are noted to be 10× the ULN. What is the most appropriate management of this adverse effect?
   A. Add milk thistle to the current regimen
   B. Change rifampin to rifabutin
   C. Discontinue ethambutol, continue all other agents
   D. Suspend all agents and reintroduce sequentially

7. The patient admits to stopping his medications after experiencing the acute spike in his liver enzymes in addition to fearing serious bleeding due to a change in the color of his urine. Which recommendation is most likely to result in a positive outcome?
   A. Change his current regimen to moxifloxacin/cycloserine/isoniazid/linezolid
   B. Obtain susceptibilities prior to reinitiating therapy
   C. Restart all therapies with twice weekly dosing in the continuation phase
   D. Restart all therapies and add bedaquiline

8. The patient is found to have positive sputum cultures at 2 months. What is the optimal (total) duration of therapy given this finding?
   A. 3 months
   B. 6 months
   C. 9 months
   D. 12 months

9. Three years after arriving in the United States the patient's son, a 32-year-old male with type 1 DM, reports to his primary care physician to have his PPD read. It is noted to be 12 mm. Which regimen is most appropriate for latent TB?
   A. Isoniazid for 9 months
   B. Isoniazid for 3 months
   C. Pyrazinamide plus rifampin for 2 months
   D. Rifampin for 4 months

10. Which supplement should be added to the patient's latent TB regimen if isoniazid is included?
    A. Ascorbic acid
    B. Cyanocobalamin (B_{12})
    C. Pyridoxine (B_6)
    D. Thiamine (B_1)

ANSWERS

1. **Explanation:** The correct answer is A. Foreign birth and immigration are considered risk factors for developing tuberculosis. Other risk factors include diabetes mellitus, prolonged use of corticosteroids, immunosuppressive therapy, injection drug use, and chronic renal failure.[1] Answer choices B and C (failure of CAP treatment and hemoptysis) are supportive in including tuberculosis in the differential diagnosis, but do not place the patient at increased risk. Answer choice D (history of COPD) has some association with tuberculosis, but is not a universally accepted risk factor.

2. **Explanation:** The correct answer is D. Confirmatory diagnosis is established by isolation of *Mycobacterium tuberculosis* from sputum or other bodily secretion. However, a positive AFB smear could also represent the presence of non-tuberculous mycobacteria (rules out answer choice A). Interferon-gamma-release assays (IGRA) and chest radiography are considered supportive diagnostic tools (rules out answer choice C). IGRAs have some utility in diagnosis but are not helpful in differentiating between latent tuberculosis and tuberculosis disease (rules out answer choice B).[2] In addition, due to the infectiousness, if active tuberculosis is in the differential diagnosis the patient should be placed in an airborne infection isolation room. Precautions can be discontinued once active tuberculosis has been ruled out, an alternative diagnosis has been established, or initiation of therapy results in three subsequent negative sputum smears.[3]

3. **Explanation:** The correct answer is D. The regimen of choice for patients with newly diagnosed pulmonary tuberculosis consists of a 4-drug intensive phase consisting of ethambutol, pyrazinamide, rifampin, and isoniazid for 2 months followed by a 2-drug continuation phase consisting of rifampin and isoniazid for 4 to 7 months.[4] Answer choice A (ethambutol plus clarithromycin) and answer choice C (rifabutin plus ethambutol) would be useful in treating non-tuberculous mycobacterial infection. Answer choice B (rifapentine and isoniazid) would be useful in treating latent tuberculosis, but not active disease.[5]

4. **Explanation:** The correct answer is A. If susceptibilities indicate lack of resistance to any of the first-line agents, ethambutol may be discontinued. Ethambutol is useful initially as it protects against rifampin resistance in the event there is unrecognized isoniazid resistance.[4]

5. **Explanation:** The correct answer is B. A well-known adverse effect of rifampin is discoloration of bodily fluids (usually a red or orange color), which is a key counseling point for patients being newly started on rifampin. In this case the patient is also on warfarin, which has a clinically significant drug–drug interaction with rifampin; however, rifampin is a CYP enzyme inducer, which would result in a lower INR and thus the urine discoloration is not a result of a drug–drug interaction but a consequence of rifampin use. Patients who require concurrent warfarin and rifampin should have close INR monitoring with adjustments being on an individual patient basis. Switching to rivaroxaban (answer choice A) would be inappropriate as this drug and other DOACs are also susceptible to drug–drug interactions with rifampin. Switching to rifapentine (answer choice C) would also not obviate the drug–drug interaction as rifapentine is also a rifamycin capable of CYP enzyme induction. Enoxaparin (answer choice D) would not interact with rifampin, but is not necessary given the INR.

6. **Explanation:** The correct answer is D. The optimal approach to reintroducing tuberculosis treatment after hepatotoxicity is not known; however, most tuberculosis programs use sequential reintroduction of drugs.[4] Because rifampin is much less likely to cause hepatotoxicity than isoniazid or pyrazinamide, it is typically restarted first followed by isoniazid. Pyrazinamide may be started 1 week after isoniazid if ALT does not increase. If rifampin and isoniazid are tolerated and hepatitis was considered severe, pyrazinamide can be assumed to be responsible and should be discontinued.[4] Answer choice A (adding milk thistle) is incorrect as this is unlikely to prevent ongoing drug-induced hepatotoxicity. Answer choice B (changing to rifabutin) is unlikely to be beneficial as clinically apparent liver injury is likely to be similar to rifampin. Answer choice C (discontinuing ethambutol) is unlikely to be helpful as the predominant toxicity with ethambutol is optic neuritis.

7. **Explanation:** The correct answer is B. When interruptions are due to an interim loss of follow-up, at the time the patient is returned to treatment, additional sputum should be obtained for repeat culture and drug susceptibility testing. Susceptibility data should be obtained prior to any change in the regimen (rules out answer choice A); moreover, adding a single agent (rules out answer choice D) to a potentially failing regimen is discouraged and likely to result in suboptimal outcomes. Twice weekly dosing (rules out answer choice C) has lesser efficacy and is more appropriate in an adherent patient.[4]

8. **Explanation:** The correct answer is C. In patients treated for 6 months, having either cavitation on chest imaging or a positive culture at completion of 2 months of therapy has been associated with rates of relapse of approximately 20% compared to 2% among patients with neither factor. For these patients, guidelines recommend extending the continuation phase with isoniazid and rifampin for an additional 3 months.[4] The other listed answer choices are either inappropriately short or long.

9. **Explanation:** The correct answer is D. The interpretation of the PPD is based on the measurement in millimeters of induration and not the degree of inflammation/erythema.

An induration of 5 mm or more is considered positive in people living with HIV, close contact with a person with active TB disease, or in persons with immunosuppression (eg, receipt of TNF blocking agents). An induration of 10 mm or more is considered positive in patients who have recently immigrated, have a history of injection drug use, and reside in high congregate settings or mycobacteriology laboratory personnel. An induration of greater than 15 mm is considered positive in any individual including those without known risk factors.[2] An induration of 12 mm in this case is suggestive of positivity due to recent immigration as well as contact with a person known to have active tuberculosis disease (father and son live in same household). The tuberculin skin test is easy to perform; however, trained personnel are needed for administration. In addition, the interpretation of the test is subject to reader variability. IGRAs, similar to the tuberculin skin test, are helpful in diagnosing infection. Moreover, IGRAs can be advantageous in certain situations including patients who have received BCG either as a vaccine or as a cancer therapy or patients unlikely to return for PPD interpretation. The utility is partially offset by cost, inconsistent test reproducibility, and increased use of laboratory resources.[2]

While there are several options for treating latent tuberculosis, adherence and tolerability should be taken into consideration when selecting any regimen. Rifampin for 4 months has a shorter treatment duration resulting in higher likelihood of adherence and better safety when compared to other listed treatment options.[6] Answer choice A (INH for 9 months) could place the patient at higher risk of peripheral neuropathy given he is diabetic. Answer choice B (INH for 3 months) is inappropriate due to the truncated duration of therapy. Answer choice C (pyrazinamide plus rifampin) is associated with higher rates of liver injury and death.

10. **Explanation:** The correct answer is C. Patients with a predisposition for neuropathy, such as those with diabetes, should receive 25 to 50 mg of pyridoxine (B_6) to prevent new onset or exacerbation of peripheral neuropathy.[5]

REFERENCES

1. Zumla A, Raviglione M, Hafner R, Fordham von Reyn C. Tuberculosis. *N Engl J Med.* 2013;368(8):745-755.
2. Lewinsohn DM, Leonard MK, LoBue PA, et al. Official American Thoracic Society/Infectious Diseases Society of America/Centers for Disease Control and Prevention clinical practice guidelines: diagnosis of tuberculosis in adults and children. *Clin Infect Dis.* 2017;64:1-33.
3. Jensen PA, Lambert LA, Iademarco MF, Ridzon R; Centers for Disease Control and Prevention. Guidelines for preventing the transmission of *Mycobacterium tuberculosis* in health-care settings. *MMWR Recomm Rep.* 2005;54(RR-17):1-141.
4. Nahid P, Dorman SE, Alipanah N, et al. Official American Thoracic Society/Centers for Disease Control and Prevention/Infectious Diseases Society of America clinical practice guidelines: treatment of drug-susceptible tuberculosis. *Clin Infect Dis.* 2016;63:147-195.
5. World Health Organization. Latent TB infection: Updated and consolidated guidelines for programmatic management, 2018. Available at http://www.who.int/tb/publications/2018/latent-tuberculosis-infection/en/. Accessed September 27, 2019.
6. Menzies D, Adjobimey M, Ruslami R, et al. Four months of rifampin or nine months of isoniazid for latent tuberculosis in adults. *N Engl J Med.* 2018;379:440-453.

INDEX